From a Safe Distance

In memory of Philip and Paddy.
Dear friends; I think of you every day.

Mais les souvenirs cheminent en nous alors que nous croyons les avoir fermement rélégués dans l'oubli.

JACQUELINE DE ROMILLY

From a Safe Distance

Suicide is Not the End of the Story

JULIA BISHOP

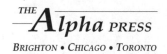

THE Alpha PRESS

BRIGHTON • CHICAGO • TORONTO

2 4 6 8 10 9 7 5 3 1

First published in 2016 by
THE ALPHA PRESS
PO Box 139
Eastbourne BN24 9BP

and in the United States of America by
THE ALPHA PRESS
Independent Publishers Group
814 N. Franklin Street, Chicago, IL 60610

and in Canada by
THE ALPHA PRESS (CANADA)

British Library Cataloguing in Publication Data
A CIP catalogue record for this book is available from the British Library.

Library of Congress Cataloging-in-Publication Data
Applied for.

Paperback ISBN 978-1-898595-70-0

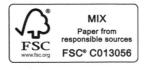

Typeset & designed by The Alpha Press, Brighton & Eastbourne.
Printed by TJ International, Padstow, Cornwall.

Contents

PART TWO: *Amends*

Author's Note

While the people, events and most of the places in the novel are fictitious (with at least two obvious exceptions, e.g. Edinburgh and Oxford), I have some real people to thank: Mum, Dad, Nick and Nev (Prof. N. G. Brown) for their constructive criticism, Fiona, Paddy for putting up with different versions and my bad moods, Donna, sorely missed, for her support in difficult times a few years ago, Steve and Claire for reading one draft along the way and Louise for proof reading and valuable comments. Dr Bob Fieldsend gave some useful insights. Finally, I thank Anthony Grahame and all at The Alpha Press for being patient with a novice.

J. D. BISHOP

Cast List of the Chief Characters

The following is not a comprehensive list; it is merely a guide.

- Main characters in the "real" world:
    Abbie, her brother Newman
    Roy Goodfield, a psychiatrist

- Others
    Matthew, Newman's son and his mother Sophie
    Sonya, Abbie's Community Psychiatric Nurse (CPN)
    Len, Abbie's uncle and stepfather

- Main characters in Abbie's book *Doors Closing:*
    Vee, her brother Jim
    Max Greenwood, a psychiatrist and his wife Helen
    Vee's mother and Uncle Ron
    Sandra, a House Manager at Squaremile

- Others
    Bella, Vee's CPN
    Simon, Max's colleague
    Jack Marshall, Senior Care Officer at Squaremile
    Squaremile's CEO, Dick Montgomery

Study me then, you who shall lovers be
At the next world, that is, at the next spring:
    For I am every dead thing,
    In whom love wrought new alchemy.
        For his art did express
A quintessence even from nothingness,
From dull privations, and lean emptiness
He ruined me, and I am re-begot
Of absence, darkness, death; things which are not.

From JOHN DONNE, *A Nocturnal upon St. Lucy's Day*

PART ONE

Amen

1

Newman Explains

How can a person have dark brown hair and not be aware of this until it starts to turn grey? Abbie was like that – more in tune with what was happening in her mind than with her appearance, or events around her. You might say my sister was a dreamer. But that didn't stop life from having an effect on her. When I read her book again over Christmas, I realised that if I tried to get it published, as I think Abbie would have liked, it would benefit from an introduction – so here it is.

Abbie wanted to tell her story. But there are parts of that story which she cannot, in reality, tell for herself. The most obvious of these is describing her own funeral, at the end of September last year.

My mother, Len and I got out of the first black car. I remember trying to focus on mundane things to avoid the reason everyone was here. Details, distractions, like how cold it was for the time of year; whether I had my gloves with me – even whether I had detected a flake of snow on the breeze. The effort I put into these preoccupations had a single purpose: to keep me ready for my speech.

Other people were arriving, looking for parking spaces, dressed for paying their respects and for warmth. I greeted a few family members who were waiting to express their sympathy. A short way off, near the chapel, I saw my mother march up to a man I didn't recognise.

'Dr Goodfield?' she asked. She sounded stressed.

The man looked uncomfortable, guilty even. He was in his fifties, of average height, with receding grey hair. A slim woman of about the same age stood next to him, holding the collar of her coat together at the neck.

'Yes, I'm Dr Goodfield. Ah, you must be Abbie's mother.'

'That's right, I am . . . ' Mum was battling tears and anger. Dr Goodfield put his hand across his mouth and bowed his head as if trying to conceal his emotion. Len held Mum's arm, murmuring something. But she went on, '*So* glad you saw fit to come today. It's a bit late for my Abbie, though.'

Turning to Len, she allowed herself to be led away. She was sobbing now, but she needed Len rather than me at the moment. Dr Goodfield. I knew the name . . . Abbie's psychiatrist, that was it.

The hearse pulled up quietly. My sister. I glanced at the coffin. But then I had to focus again on simple things, divert my attention: the footsteps of the people moving towards the chapel, the first wet, brown leaves underfoot, and putting my gloves into the pocket of my overcoat. We took our seats at the front. My speech was in my inside pocket.

About twenty people had assembled in the chapel. The coffin was brought in, to quiet organ music. Then the priest spoke the usual comforting phrases, his voice coming out of the depths of this dark, old-fashioned building. After the single hymn, there were sombre prayers. Then it was my turn. It seemed to take me a very long time to reach the lectern, in the brittle silence which enveloped me.

'I am Newman, Abbie's brother.' I felt a tightening in my throat. 'Most of you know that already.' A few moments passed before I could continue, and I was aware that my piece of paper was shaking. 'A terrible illness, a long struggle, is over.' I swallowed. 'Abbie was a very private person. I remember how, when we were children, she would spend hours in her room . . . ' I hesitated, then went on, 'She would spend hours reading, or writing poetry. She used to win competitions!' I felt this moment of lightness die on my lips. 'She carried on writing to the end. To finish, I would like to read a poem she wrote a couple of years ago, which is dedicated to her psychiatrist.' Despite the groan from my mother, and a vague sense of being tactless, I felt I had to finish what I had started. I cleared my throat. 'It's called, "The Man in the Office".

> "It is easy to forget her –
> The nurse by the door – as
> Your shoes are all I can see,
> Your chair in front of mine.
>
> You cross your legs, waiting, as if
> Time has no meaning. You speak gently, but
> Can't you hear the crashing waves?
> We are not in the same storm."'

Returning to my seat, I felt a sense of relief. All that could be heard for a short while was the creaking of wooden pews and one or two coughs. I could not bring myself to look at my mother, as my own grief was enough. Nor did I pay attention to the priest's closing words; all I could do was stare at the coffin as the curtains closed, aware as the finality pierced my being.

Outside, I wanted to catch Dr Goodfield, who was just getting into his car. He looked surprised when I called out to him.

'Thank you for coming, doctor. I hope – '

'– Roy: call me Roy, please. And this is my wife, Madeleine.' She was already in the passenger seat, but leant forward to say hello. She had an attractive smile.

'Will we see you at the pub?' I asked.

'No, I'm afraid we've got to get back.' He looked anxious.

'Ah, I see.' I hesitated. 'Roy, can I come and see you, to . . . talk about things?' Seeing his pallor, I added, 'Please don't think I blame you. I mean, I'm not angry.'

He seemed to respond to this reassurance. 'Well, yes. If you want to talk. I mean, yes, of course.' He fumbled for his wallet. 'Here's my card. Oh, actually – I've got something of Abbie's you should have, so it would be a good idea to meet. Give me a call when you're ready.'

I turned, with the intention of going to comfort my mother, but everyone had gone.

I have always hated going up in the attic. I don't like spending any length of time in the same room as cobwebs and seldom used things. On this occasion, I wanted to find some old photographs as well as getting the Christmas decorations down, aiming to grab everything and leave without delay.

I found the boxes I was looking for, and handed them through the hatch to Matthew. Then I noticed that lying on top of the last one was something else: the book Abbie had written, in a thick brown folder, already dusty. I was ashamed to realise that I had forgotten all about it. Crouching under the lamp, I flicked through the typescript, noticing several crossings-out and handwritten changes. I suddenly remembered the day she had given me the book to read, back at the start of the summer, and how I had skimmed through it without really understanding. I should try again now, I thought. Her death had changed things.

In the dim light, I noticed Abbie's original title: *Doors Closing* which, when I thought for a moment, I realised was the voice of the hospital lifts.

'Come on Dad! There's still one more lot of stuff to come yet!' Matthew was still waiting. 'And did you find the photos?'

If I was aiming for publication on Abbie's behalf, a less depressing, more positive title would have to be found. I would give it some thought. As I passed the last box down to Matthew and took the folder with me, I knew that questions were about to be asked. I was right.

'Dad, are you ever going to tell me about Auntie Abbie? I mean, I think I'm old enough to understand. I know what happened to Mum, so can it be any worse than that?'

We sat in the lounge. Matthew began opening the boxes and stretched out a length of tinsel.

'Yes, I think you probably are old enough, and I do intend

to tell you – I hadn't forgotten, son. It's just that I don't really know the whole story myself yet.'

'What, even after all this time?'

'Well, she only died a few months ago; I'm still finding things out.'

'Is that hers, that folder you're holding?'

'Yes.'

'Can I look at it?' Matthew came towards me.

My son deserved a proper explanation, but not right then. And it was not going to be straightforward.

'As soon as I have the full picture, I'll tell you all about her. Then you can look at this. But I've got one or two photos of her. Will that do for now?'

I was used to making this kind of "when-should-he-be-allowed-to" decision on my own, since his mother's death when Matthew was only three. He seemed satisfied with my conditions and studied the photos.

An introduction should set the scene and explain a few things. In her book, Abbie has two aims. Firstly, she wants to tell her story, which she felt unable to express in any other way. And it *needed* to be expressed, in order to render it less threatening to Abbie herself. Talking about her illness was difficult for her, as I know first hand. While I accept that it wasn't like discussing what to wear, she seemed to think that talking somehow tended to invite criticism and prejudice.

So instead of talking, she wrote; in this way, she avoided an immediate challenge. It gave her the chance to put down the facts and the chance to be *believed*. Being believed and being accepted were vital. Not being believed or accepted made her feel suffocated. I don't know what that feels like.

Once the thoughts, the experiences were liberated by being written down, they might reach others as well. By doing this, she could both convey her story and correct any assumptions we might have made. It was just sad she had to die first.

Her second aim is to expose and deal with an injustice which affected her profoundly. I am no philosopher or psychologist, but I know perfectly well that our experiences change us, even if we want to forget the bad times. I know that especially from losing my wife. At the same time, I admit to having had great difficulty in understanding both the nature and the effects of my sister's illness, which may have meant that I was sometimes less than sympathetic. I couldn't accept that the thing would keep coming back, so I couldn't understand why Abbie didn't just go out and find a new job, when she was fit and well. Why wasn't she making any effort? It wasn't her usual approach to a challenge. I was keen to get her to justify her behaviour. She mentioned "stigma", and having "a history", but I thought she was looking for excuses, even making the most of it.

But then what do I know? If it wasn't that bad, why did Abbie kill herself? She's not here any more to explain things to me, but her death has rendered my assumptions, my irritation, trivial. There is a tendency for people to be less sympathetic towards those they are close to. I come up against that every day at work. It must be because emotional attachment brings with it a kind of "expectation of competence". And that works both ways.

If I have learnt anything from Abbie's death, it is that, family or not, if we deride or punish, then we are just as much to blame as this destructive illness. While it might seem to have a mind of its own, an illness, however, has neither mercy nor conscience.

It was one of those bright, cold January days when the wind parts your hair in unexpected places. I was no stranger to the hospital because of my work, but as I was early for my appointment with Roy Goodfield, I stood looking down over Howcester, its grey and red buildings strewn across the valley.

The steep hospital road was lined with short bushes which strained in the wind. It was not long before I decided to go indoors. This building, the Porteblanche Unit, was the newest part of the hospital and a marvel of architectural design. Outside the main entrance the hard standing was protected by a roof extension for people arriving in bad weather. The automatic doors opened on to a spacious reception area, which had been refurbished since my last visit, with comfortable chairs, small tables, posters and racks of leaflets on the walls. About half a dozen people were waiting. At the far end, to the right, was the desk, sealed like a bank window.

'Hello, Newman.' Roy had come in just behind me. I realised how much taller I was than him.

'Oh, hello, Roy.' We shook hands. 'Cold, isn't – '

'– Hey, it's you, fuckin' Goodfield. I'm in 'ere again 'cos of you, you bastard!' The loud voice which had interrupted me belonged to a young man who was now walking towards us in determined fashion. He was unshaven, with long greasy hair and a hole in his green sweater.

There was a sound of vacated chairs as the other people, anxious, gathered by the opposite wall. I noticed that the receptionist was making a call. The young man was standing quite close to us now, breathing heavily and trembling. Moments later, two large male nursing assistants burst through the double doors to the left of reception and came over to escort the patient back to his ward. He did not resist. In fact he began to weep, and walked quietly away with the nurses.

Roy seemed unperturbed, keeping his dignity, in his neat black cashmere overcoat, all the while clutching a fat brown folder under his arm. He had a quiet word with the receptionist, then we made our way through the same double doors, Roy using his key card, down to his office.

'Good journey?' Roy asked.

'Fine thanks.' Our voices echoed and the heavy fire doors creaked. 'Thanks for seeing me.'

'Not at all. I just had to go out to the car for something. Been here all day, but I couldn't expect you to find my office, so we timed it perfectly.' He smiled.

A smell of disinfectant mixed with tobacco pervaded the top corridor, full of sunlight. After two more sets of doors, the sound of our footsteps was suddenly muffled as we reached the carpeted area. As Roy opened his office door, I saw a young woman sitting reading a document. She stood up, and Roy introduced us.

'This is Sonya, Abbie's CPN. Newman, Abbie's brother.' We shook hands and a silver bracelet slid down her arm. She had thick black hair and large, thin loop earrings. Her dark eyes showed compassion for the loss of my sister.

Roy wanted to explain his behaviour in reception.

'That business back there – it might have looked callous', he said, placing the brown folder next to his rather scruffy briefcase on the end of the desk and taking off his coat, 'but my policy is never to engage with a patient when they first come in, until they have been assessed by the nursing staff – and given some meds if necessary.'

'I see. Sounds fair enough. I mean, not callous at all.'

I took off my coat and scarf, draped them over a spare chair and we sat down.

'I'm not stopping', Sonya said. 'I just had to pop in to give Roy some notes after he'd seen his last patient. Then he said you were coming, so I thought I'd stay and meet you.'

It was a functional, plain room. There was no couch, as people imagine; just reasonably comfortable chairs, magnolia walls, a computer desk with swivel chair tucked away, shelving above the main desk with drawers, and a small low table in the middle where Carol, Roy's secretary, placed a tray of coffee and biscuits. This was a welcome sight. The door clicked shut behind her.

'So,' Sonya asked, 'what do you do for a living?'

'I'm a social worker', I replied, 'over in Oxford.'

'Oh, yes. Abbie did say, but I'd forgotten. So you must be used to hospitals and care homes.'

'Well, yes, but each has its own character.'

'Have you ever been to the residential centre called Squaremile?' Sonya glanced at Roy, who sat quietly in front of the main desk, then looked earnestly at me, leaning forward slightly, both hands in her lap.

'Only once, for work.'

'What did you think of it?' She leant forward to pick up her cup.

I chose my words carefully. 'Well, I didn't know what to make of it. Have you got any connection with the place?'

'No, it's just a coincidence that Abbie worked there, so I visited quite regularly.'

'Yes, of course.' I suddenly felt guilty.

'And I know what a hard time she had. They were really rough on her. Huge place, though, isn't it? Roy works there one day a week, don't you?'

Roy nodded.

Then, with a short gasp, Sonya realised the time. 'Oh, but look, I must get going now, and let you both talk. Bye for now.' She picked up her belongings and left.

'So how can I help?' asked Roy.

'There are two things I just can't get my head round.'

'Go on.'

'The first one is obvious: why did Abbie kill herself?'

'It has to do with being bipolar – or as they used to call it, manic depressive. You know I can't discuss Abbie specifically, but she is typical. Some people reach a point where they feel they simply can't bear it any longer. That's it in a nutshell. Of course I can't begin to imagine what that *feels* like but it's a fact.'

Roy stood up and walked over to the window. Neither of us spoke for a few moments. Then he returned to his seat opposite me, his clear blue eyes and silver hair catching the low afternoon sunlight. He cleared his throat. A subtle change had occurred in his expression, which I couldn't account for, unless what Abbie had written was true? His voice was slightly hoarse too. 'What was the second thing on your mind?'

'It was . . . well, it doesn't really matter, now she's gone, but I could never understand why she gave up looking for work.'

'Before I answer that, can I ask *you* a question?' Roy appeared to have recovered now.

'OK.'

'Was it important for *you* that she had a job?'

'Um, only for her well-being and sense of worth. I would feel happy if she was happy.'

'I see. No other reason?'

'Not that I can think of, no.'

Roy smiled an enigmatic smile which was slightly unnerving. He crossed his legs. 'Sorry. Old habits and all that. Anyway, as for why Abbie, and many others, stop looking for work, there are two main reasons. Firstly, there is the dragon called stigma. At the time when Abbie was applying for jobs, she knew she had to declare her illness – .'

' – What d'you mean, *had* to? How would they know, if Abbie was OK most of the time?' I could feel my indignation rising.

'Because, Newman, if she didn't declare it and got the job, she could've been sacked on the spot if they found out or when she got ill again! Notice I say *when*, not *if*!' Roy was quite agitated. He uncrossed his legs and placed a hand on each thigh. 'That's one way in which stigma operates. It was a case of "catch 22", because if she declared it, and they interviewed her – because of the so-called anti-discrimination laws – all the employer had to do was find a different, bogus reason for not offering her the job, while everybody knew full well what the real reason was. Nowadays, at least people are not obliged to declare their disability in advance. Mind you, it used to be even worse: until a few years ago, a medical questionnaire with the application form often made sure there was no interview at all. "Weeding them out" was a phrase

I heard my patients use more than once.'

We sat in silence for a moment.

'I wasn't properly aware of all this', I ventured. 'You must have known quite a few people who had these difficulties with work.'

Roy smiled his answer. More a grimace really. He was calmer, showing only the last traces of indignation. 'No, people aren't aware, unless they're faced with it themselves', he went on, 'like a lot of things in life. For some people, only their *own* pain is real.' He paused, and sighed. 'Another point I wanted to make follows on from this: the situation I've described is not designed to inspire confidence. So no matter what your qualifications or suitability, if you knew this is what you were up against, you just wouldn't see any point in applying. It's a perfectly sensible, logical reaction – a means of self-preservation. Rejection hurts; once bitten, as the saying goes. Add to that the uncertainty of the illness itself, the competition for jobs which exists for *everybody*, and the passing years giving you a history, with progressively less and less chance of employment, and there's your answer. And in the end, whatever the current rules, you see, you are still going to be asked, "Why did you leave your last job?" and "What have you been doing for the last umpteen years?"'

'Well, I kind of worked that bit out, but . . . ' I looked down at the empty cups and remaining biscuits, remembering with some pain how I had kept on at Abbie to apply for jobs. Then: 'Roy, you said *when* she was ill again. Why not *if* ?'

'Because it's in the very nature of bipolar disorder. People can be in remission for years, but in nine cases out of ten there will always be another episode. That's one cause of suicide, I'm sorry to say. A lethal combination of uncertainty and terror.'

'My last question is, why did Abbie have to take medication when she was well?'

'It's to lessen the severity of future attacks, or lengthen the time between.'

'Oh, I see.'

There was a knock at the door.

'Come in!' Roy called. It was Carol, to collect the tray. When she had left, Roy changed the subject, to my relief. 'Well, I mentioned at the funeral that I had something to give you.' He turned and picked up the thick brown folder with both hands, placing it on his lap. 'It's Abbie's book. Did you know about it?'

'Yes. I have a copy and I've read it.'

Roy looked a little sheepish, a little disconcerted at what

I might have read. 'I'm afraid I haven't – yet. I've been in two minds. I was going to give it back to you, but –'

'– Roy, I think you should read it, because whether it's all true or not, I believe you play a very important part in it.'

My introduction to Abbie's – or should I say Vee's – book is nearly complete. I might still change a few more names in her story, but for the moment I have little more to say.

I plan to include my introduction in the version for publication. Now it is time for Abbie (Vee) to tell her story, *Doors Closing*. You will notice that her imagined funeral bears an uncanny resemblance to my description of the event. She begins by exploring what might have happened when "Max" has to make a decision.

2

A Toe in the Water

"Why are they being so nice to me? I am angry because I am failing, so why aren't they angry with me too? Then I see it. The white door is swinging open, the padlock hanging by a curved metal finger, and a black tunnel appears; I can hear the echo of rows of black doors closing sharply along it, like an old train about to leave. A voice repeats that I am useless. The white door, the whole building, seems to be moving slightly, up and down, and getting larger, filling the world . . .

"Someone is asking me questions in a quiet place with soft chairs. I try to answer, but my voice is slow and old . . . An arm points to a bed in a small room. I am a grey slab floating on a dark sea".

Max switched off his bedside light. He had brought Vee's book home, but he had not opened it until now.

Helen murmured softly beside him as he made himself comfortable.

'Max?' she said quietly in the dark.

'Darling?'

'What's that you were reading?'

'Oh, nothing. Just . . . work.'

The black cars made their dignified approach along the drive which led to the crematorium. A handful of people waited outside as the afternoon sun began to wane. It makes sense that as you grow older, you go to more funerals. But this one was too soon; Vee was too young. For Max, she had been the one; it was the first time he had ever fallen in love, many years ago. Now he would never see her again. Why, he wondered, do the most profound thoughts often sound so stupid and trite?

At the moment the important thing was to stay calm; Helen knew nothing of the part Vee had played in her husband's life, so his grief had to be appropriate, moderate – above all, under control. As far as Helen was concerned, he had only ever been Vee's doctor, for the last year or so.

People emerged from vehicles, straightening their clothing. An elderly couple got out of one car and made their way towards Max.

'Dr Greenwood?' the woman asked.

'Yes. You must be Vee's mother.'

'That's right. Thank you for coming. It's a bit late for Vee though. 'Here, take it.' She thrust a large envelope into his hands. 'It's addressed to you, so you might as well have it.' She turned away quickly.

He was not surprised at her behaviour: it reawakened the guilt he was trying to ignore. The great bolus of guilt which lay on his chest like a ball of lead. Helen's arm tightened in his and she gave him a worried look. Mrs Gates and her tall thin husband were talking to another couple now, his arm round her shoulder. Max hadn't wanted to come here today, because of the private fear of an excess of grief. But Helen had persuaded him. He'd tried every excuse that morning: he didn't feel up to it; they were going to a party in the evening; a funeral was not his idea of a day out, and so on. She had been concerned by his behaviour, but decided not to say anything; she knew her husband. But Max, thinking that saying goodbye would probably be the last thing he could do for Vee, gave in to Helen; she needed him. The fact was that she was there not just as his wife, but as the only representative from Squaremile, who seemed to have turned their collective back on recent events.

While they waited outside, he thought about grief. People grieve in different ways; a pattern is not always evident, despite the neat stages identified by psychologists. Grief can be unpredictable, making people behave out of character. In a case like Vee's, however, he knew that close family often start by looking for someone to blame. Mrs Gates only saw in him the doctor who hadn't prevented her daughter from killing herself.

How would he feel if he lost one of his children? Impossible to say. But he did know that most parents want to hold their children, protect them from the world. At the same time, they recognise that this isn't possible either – not for ever, anyway. He remembered when Grace had meningitis. He didn't know if it was God he had to thank when she recovered, just as he didn't know if there were such things as souls that lived on after death, except perhaps in people's memories, where they would eventually die in turn. Old graves have no visitors in grief.

There was a movement towards the chapel, so they filed in and took their places, standing while Mrs Gates and her companion passed to the front, with a younger man whom he thought must be Jim. Finally, in silence, the coffin was brought in.

After the single hymn, there were sombre prayers, then the younger man at the front was invited to stand at the lectern.

'I am Jim Gates, Vee's brother.' His deep voice faltered a little. He coughed, the edge of his trembling paper just visible. He managed to get to the end of his notes, finishing with one of Vee's poems, which Max recognised, with a lurch of his stomach. It was about him. It made him feel uncomfortable, as if it was too private. He flexed his fingers deep in his gloves and Helen glanced at him. At least it was short.

Jim returned to his seat. Max noticed a late butterfly, trying to escape at a high window. He did not pay attention to what the priest said next, but then Vee's coffin began to move away from them, the curtain closed and he felt a sudden and terrible stab of sorrow which fixed him to the spot for a few moments. Max and Helen didn't wait around long after that. They were not family.

On the last day of the year Max was spending time in his attic office at home while Helen clattered about downstairs. He had a feeling she was making him a birthday cake. He didn't really want to celebrate though, to be honest. He desperately wanted to talk about Vee and let out all his grief, but he recognised at the same time how dangerous this could be, so he wouldn't have a drink if Helen offered him one, birthday or no birthday. Sadly, avoiding the subject could easily turn into avoiding Helen. The guilt and pain would not go away and he didn't know what to do about it.

Finding a time to open the envelope given to him by Mrs Gates at the funeral had been tricky too, and Helen knew he was keeping something from her – which he was, of course. It was natural that she should be curious about the contents of this envelope and why Mrs Gates had given it to him. He dreaded the possibility of a confrontation, and was preoccupied with finding a way out. Of course, he didn't want to cause Helen unnecessary pain either.

The envelope contained a letter and Vee's last diary. The letter asked him to read her book, if he hadn't already done so. He'd had *Doors Closing* since their last appointment, but had told himself he didn't have time. And then there was that strange remark . . . The diary was written in a blunter style than the book and was quite disturbing; he would keep it hidden behind the computer monitor.

He was trying to keep a record of events, in case there were any tricky questions to answer: there would definitely be an inquest into her death. Even without this motive, he found the act of writing helpful. When he'd seen Vee for the last time back in August, he'd judged her to be euthymic, with no formal thought disorder. In other words, she gave no cause for concern, despite having lost her job in June. There was no indication of what was to happen so soon afterwards. It proves how quickly this illness can take hold. He had half expected some kind of outburst from Vee, as he had instructed Bella, Vee's Community Psychiatric Nurse, to let her know he was retiring. Bella did mention that Vee had been upset, but at her appointment with him, she appeared to have only one thing on her mind: handing over the book.

'Max?' Helen was on the stairs.

'I'll be down in a minute.'

He tried to imagine the final scene at Vee's flat. According to Bella, Vee's CPN for several years, she arrives in Cressington expecting to meet Vee as usual. Getting no answer, Bella decides to ask the neighbours if they have seen Vee or spoken to her recently. The only person she can find is a young girl, who shrugs and pulls a face to start with, but then jumps when she remembers Vee gave her a key, as she says, "for cat-feeding and emergencies". She runs upstairs to get it. Then, with some trepidation, and the girl standing big-eyed behind her, Bella unlocks the front door. She finds Vee lying on the bed with the cat curled up beside her. She had timed it for Bella to find her.

Going back to their August appointment, he could see in his mind's eye the way Vee walked into the room hugging the thick folder in a plastic bag, her eyes showing what he interpreted as a fear of being rejected, her coat wet on the shoulders. She said she wasn't sure if the book was finished, he remembered, but didn't think she could do much more to it. She did not appear triumphant after all her work. She was, however, quite insistent that he read it, saying as she left, "You'll know what to do". Although she was being mysterious, he'd assumed at the time that she wanted him to check it through, but now he suspected there was more to it than that.

He would "know what to do". What did she mean? And what effect could he possibly have on anything, or anyone, now? People at Squaremile, for example, had probably forgotten all about Vee and the damage they did to her. Out of sight, out of mind. He knew Helen had worked with Vee for a short time at Squaremile, but she'd never mentioned anything.

Compounding his guilt regarding her suicide, he was ashamed to admit that, four months on, he'd only opened the book the night before, in bed, and even then, he hadn't started at the beginning. The answers to his questions must be in that folder, but did he really want to find out? He felt daunted.

'How long are you going to be? It's your favourite.'

'Not long; give me two minutes.'

As a way of avoiding reading it, a way of trying to set a boundary between the professional and the personal, he thought Vee's folder should now be returned to the Gates family and the whole matter laid to rest along with its author. Perhaps what she wanted from him was too difficult; even if he read the book, there was a chance he'd be no further forward. But now he was making excuses again. He slammed his fist down on the desk. The book would just have to be returned, that was that. The situation was intolerable.

But examining his emotions required honesty: he had to face up to the fact that reading a book by someone who might once have been his wife, knowing the outcome, demanded courage. And he was a coward in matters of the heart. Besides, with his retirement approaching, he wanted to wind down, not take on any new projects. Finding he was trying to justify his behaviour only made him more aware that he was on shaky ground; the simple truth required no embellishment: he was afraid to read *Doors Closing* because he did not want Vee's words to reawaken something that could cause him even more pain.

There. He put the folder in his very tatty briefcase, which had given years of service, ready to take back to work, where he would keep it for the time being, and went downstairs to his wife.

'Happy Birthday, darling!' She kissed him and they sat down. She had gone to a lot of trouble. She made him blow out the single candle on his cake and he felt himself relax in the warmth of her company. As he looked at her across the table, her short dark hair framing the softness of her face, her eyes smiling as she laughed at a feeble joke, he felt glad, convinced after all that his life was as it should be. We only get one chance, he thought, and regrets can weigh us down.

He would give Vee's book back. Making that decision eased the pain a little, temporarily, but a degree of curiosity remained. He needed to talk to someone. But whom could he trust?

3

Simon

Often the only way to relieve the guilt people feel about something important is by taking some kind of action. Reluctantly, he had to admit that this applied to him. Vee had known this too.

Max carried on writing down his thoughts to do with Vee at the hospital after work, during his last days at Porteblanche. Predictably, staying late did not make him popular with Helen. A voice broke into his thoughts. It was Simon, the colleague he would probably choose to confide in.

'Hi, Max! What are you doing still here at this hour?'

'Oh, it's a long story. But I could ask you the same question.'

How would he broach the subject? He had known Simon for some years and he trusted his professional judgement, even if the man was possessed of a frantic determination to see the lighter side of everything. But to his credit, Simon never minced his words. He still had the enthusiasm and looks of a junior doctor, but the wisdom of a fellow consultant. He was between five and ten years younger than Max, heavily built, with blond hair, looking a bit like Boris Johnson.

'Drink?' Simon asked.

'OK, but I'll have to ring the wife.'

Simon was divorced. Standing in the doorway in his dark overcoat, collar and tie and polished black shoes and carrying a neat black briefcase, he made Max feel scruffy in his brown cords and check shirt. Simon resembled a character from a 1960s British TV police drama, Max thought, and it occurred to him that the young doctor's "uniform" had moved back in time from the beige chinos and blue shirts of ten years ago.

While Max rang Helen, Simon went back into his office next door and returned with the latest edition of *Shrink* magazine in his hand. Max finished his call and put his phone in his very tatty briefcase. Simon pointed out this month's amusing story in the magazine, which Max had read. They both laughed. Max grabbed his coat.

They went in convoy to a pub on the way to Okebury, where Simon lived, hoping they would not be recognised. Max noticed that Simon's car was looking a bit elderly. Their headlights scoured white semi-circles on the building as they drove on to the flattened gravel. It began to snow. The pub was packed; they plunged into a room filled with the deafening roar of competing conversations, punctuated by shrieks of laughter. For a second he thought of the Smoking Room at Porteblanche. But the behaviour of these people could be put down to alcohol rather than psychosis. Luckily, a group was just leaving, so the two men pushed their way into the alcove. Someone slopped his drink on Simon's coat: 'Sorry mate!' Because they were driving, they made one drink last forty minutes. Gone were the student days of carefree and competitive inebriation. Simon paid, but it took him ten minutes to get served. When he finally got back, he demanded to know what the "long story" was which had kept Max late at work, so Max attempted to explain. He would have to, if he wanted to pick Simon's brains.

'Hang on; you say you went to her funeral?' Simon looked worried. 'But why?'

'Helen wanted to go because of working at Squaremile. But if you must know, there is another reason, which made things difficult for me, actually. I knew Vee years ago, before she was ill.'

'Knew her – what, in the Biblical sense?'

Max looked him straight in the face. Simon's light brown eyes glinted with mischief as he took a mouthful of beer.

Max found he was strangely calm, but he still had to raise his voice above the noise.

'It was all a long time ago. Of course, Helen knows nothing about this – and I want to try and keep it that way.' He told Simon some of the story.

At first, Simon's face lit up, but then it turned sour: 'Bugger me, Max! She must have really been something. Huh, wouldn't catch me doing all that for a woman,' he added, with a flippancy close to cynicism. 'Nearly giving up a job? So,' he went on, 'let me get this straight. Now, from beyond the grave, she commands you to read a book she was writing, which probably contains adult material about you. She also seems to expect something else from you. What did she say? "You'll know what to do". What the hell is that all about?' Simon frowned, stiffening his neck backwards.

'Sounds crazy, I know.'

Max told him how Vee became his patient years after their relationship had ended, and about the way she had been treated at work. Working at Squaremile one day a week allowed him only a glimpse of life there. Max was aware that the conditions in the pub were not right for asking advice nor, for that matter, for talking at all. The noise was tremendous, so subtlety would have been impossible. And in the end, he wasn't sure if Simon was the right person. He decided to bide his time; he'd said enough.

Simon put his large hands on the table as he spoke, one each side of his pint glass. 'I know what it is. You're worried because you feel guilty. Am I right, or am I right?' He lifted his head, nodded slightly with certainty and gave Max a quizzical look. Then, lowering his voice and leaning towards his colleague, serious for once: 'Hey! You mustn't let guilt about her suicide eat you up! It happens.' He was almost gentle. 'Have you got a date for the inquest?'

'No, not yet.'

He drew back, both arms out in front of him on the table. 'When did she die?'

'September.'

'So it can't be far off. Then you can start to forgive yourself.' Simon folded his arms and went on, 'Now then: are you going to read this book, because I think, my friend, that if you do, you'll find out what she was on about, what she wanted you to do. And from what you've told me, I would guess that it has something to do with that Squaremile place.'

Simon was making it all sound so straightforward, Max thought.

'But Max, if I'm right, it boils down to whether you want to take on what could be a difficult job, tackling an established organisation. Personally, I wouldn't want to know, but I didn't know Vee the way you did. Seriously though Max, there are other things to consider: your marriage, your reputation – your health, even. And do you intend to do Vee's bidding, whatever it may be, on your own?'

Max shook his head and finished his pint.

Simon continued. 'There are practicalities. 'Oh, come on, Max! Admit it! It's guilt pure and simple. Do you really want to let guilt take you down this unknown road?'

Max had had enough. 'Come on, let's get out of here. I can hardly hear myself think. I didn't think it would be this busy in here. What's more, you've worn me out.'

Simon laughed out loud. 'Time to move on, Max. Time to move on.'

If he decided to speak to Simon again about Vee, he would see him the next day, and the conditions would be better. The office at the Porteblanche Unit could be draughty, especially at this time of year, but at least it was quieter than the pub. Max didn't get as many external phonecalls as he used to, but some were still put through to him, such as the occasional invitation to give a talk to some self-help group or other. He didn't have so many patients to see either, in or out, now the majority had been reassigned. He had, however, reviewed the young man with the hole in his jumper who'd come in the other day; he'd calmed down, but was still resentful at having been sectioned.

Max heard his colleagues leaving one by one, and the

sound of a vacuum cleaner in the corridor. A particularly strong gust of January wind blew and the lights went out. The hospital generator kicked in after a few seconds. The door was ajar; hearing someone cough outside, he guessed who was there.

'Come in!'

'Working late again?' Simon came in, smiling.

'Hmm. Simon. What is somebody of your age doing hanging around draughty psych departments after hours? Haven't you got a home to go to?'

Simon was slow to answer. 'Well no, actually. It was repossessed. The recession and all that.' He looked uncharacteristically vulnerable.

'Oh, I'm sorry. That was tactless of me.'

'You weren't to know. My son and I are dossing down at my brother's for the time being, but it's difficult because I don't like to be in the way too much and cramp his style: he's got a new girlfriend.'

Max was preoccupied. He picked up the handful of papers he had just printed off and tapped them together on the desk. 'D'you know something?' he said, sitting in an armchair. 'I've realised what I need to do.'

'What's that then?' Simon sat with one buttock on the desk, one foot in mid air.

'There's no reason why I shouldn't tell you the whole story. It's just that –'

'– Max, what are you on about?'

Max took a deep breath. 'What I've realised is that the person who really needs to know everything is Helen. Please don't be offended, but . . . I'm just a coward, you see. It's not her feelings I think I'm sparing, but my own. But then that's not true either, is it? If I told her, I wouldn't feel so anxious to avoid her. And several things have happened to make her suspicious – God only knows what she's thinking now. She's probably feeling pretty sad. I know I would feel left out if I thought she had secrets.'

'Max, this is all very well but, pangs of conscience aside, do you want to jeopardise your marriage over an old flame, who's dead anyway? And when you haven't even been unfaithful? You didn't – I mean, after Helen, did you?'

'You mean, have sex with a patient? Of course not. I may be retiring soon, but that doesn't give me an excuse to break the rules. No, I haven't been unfaithful to Helen, with Vee or anyone else. Vee was . . . a long time ago.' Max looked at Simon, stood up and slipped the new sheets of paper into his briefcase. Simon moved to a chair.

'Forgive me for saying this Simon, but what you said just now about jeopardising my marriage: you've got it the wrong way round,' said Max. 'I think I'd be jeopardising my marriage if I *didn't* tell Helen. My discomfort and her suspicion combine to make an elephant in the room.'

'How about if I advised you *not* to read Vee's book then? That way, the discomfort and suspicion won't last because they don't go too deep. I agree that you can't leave things as they are, but if you read the book, you might be asking for trouble. It's easier to sort out a small problem than deal with what Vee might have written. You have no guarantee it's positive! If she was ill, she could've written anything about you!'

Standing by the desk, Max thought for a moment. 'If that's the case, I think I'm better off knowing about it, especially as I don't know who else has read it, apart from her brother. Wouldn't you prefer to know what someone's written about you – something that might have been in circulation before you even knew it existed?'

'Well, if you put it like that, I suppose so.'

Max picked up his case and coat. 'I've had an idea,' he announced. 'I want to be honest with Helen. And I want to get her involved. Thanks, Simon, but I know where to start.'

While a definite plan of action eluded him at this stage, he continued recording his thoughts at home. This had become not only a routine but a necessity; he realised it was keeping Vee alive for him. He would find the right time to talk to

Helen and he would read the book. This decision made him feel more confident.

He hadn't told Simon or Helen about Jim's visit to Porteblanche that week, and how he had been persuaded to keep his copy of the book rather than give it back to Vee's family. Jim had told Max that he played a "very important part" in the book; this was intriguing. While talking to Simon, he had realised that Helen was the obvious, perfect person to help him – that is, of course, if things worked out– because Simon was right: he would not be able to act alone.

The light in the attic room changes. Max finds himself in a lecture theatre, addressing a group of medical students about the effects of suicide on hospital personnel. He is in a spotlight, on the platform. Their faces are in darkness; all he can see is a rough arc of light, which moves according to who is speaking, at the top of each head, lighting up hair as if there is a projector behind them. He begins: –

"When someone dies like this, the people involved in her care cannot help feeling guilty. We always think we should have seen the signs and acted more quickly".

"But we can't see into their mind, can we, so what can we do?" A student in the front row blurts out.

"Exactly. If someone is really determined to do some-thing, there is very little anyone can do about it. Criticism from outside is not helpful, nor is hindsight. They do nothing to assuage guilt. We have to absolve ourselves if we are to continue, in order to give the best care possible to our other patients. I have never experienced – and I hope I never do – the kind of difficulties, the mindset that leads to suicidal thoughts, so I cannot hope to appreciate how a patient was feeling on a daily basis".

The lecture theatre fades, the light returns to normal. But he still has a vague sense that Vee is watching him. There were plenty of reasons why he should *not* go on with some kind of investigation, especially with regard to confidentiality: he hoped he would not be put in an awkward position regarding Vee. On the other hand, Vee did choose to make aspects of her life public in the first place by writing *Doors Closing*.

4

Turning a page

It was his last day at Porteblanche. He had to remind Helen of that, when she started to ask him again what he had been doing working so late. She'd had to throw away his dinner last night and wasn't happy. At breakfast he pointed out that from now on, she would be desperate to get him *out* of the house rather than back in it.

The last ever ward round: Max felt a kind of excitement. Wearing a dark, smart suit for a change, he went down the stairs and reached the long, spacious corridor, a light green tube lit from the right by a pale afternoon sun. The echo of his footsteps as he made his way to the acute wards filled him with a sense of the importance of this moment in his life. He would probably only get to see two or three patients today who were ready for discharge, as his colleagues were already looking after the others.

He was surprised at how his last day had crept up and was here, now. As he entered the first ward, Simon was just leaving.

'You won't disappear at five, will you?' the younger man said quietly.

'Why?' Max raised his eyebrows in feigned innocence.

'Well, you never know, there might be drinks in it,' he replied, tapping the side of his nose and heading for the door.

'More than one?'

Simon grinned as he went out into the corridor. When the rounds on both acute wards were over, Max had cards and good wishes from the nurses, then champagne and gifts in the largest office upstairs.

He was frogmarched up there by two nursing assistants, who announced: "We found this unsavoury character lurking on the wards!" A cheer went up. But because of the impending work concerning Vee, he didn't feel as if he was really retiring.

The office had looked bare as he shut the door for the last time, but he knew that a fresh young doctor would be moving in before long. He wished whoever it was the best of luck; he had seen a lot of changes during his career, some of them not for the better. The textbook he had used when training, by Slater and Roth, had emphasised the dignity of patients and inculcated respect for them in their suffering. Nowadays, he felt, basic kindness was sometimes forgotten, replaced by reliance on medication.

He brought the fat folder home again of course, along with three boxes of books from his shelves. Helen's photo sat on the top of one box, smiling up at him as he took it to the car. One of the nurses carried the other boxes out for him, but at home, Helen wanted the whole lot put up in the attic office straight away. He was pretty out of breath when he'd done that. He was not as fit as he might have been. Helen had on more than one occasion suggested he go to the Well Man clinic, but he never seemed to get round to it.

Helen had taken a few days off to coincide with Max's retirement, but that day she was meeting a friend. All the same, as expected, she was desperate to know what he was up to.

'It's just that, well, I thought the work you were doing in the evening would stop once you finished at Porteblanche! What is that great fat folder, anyway?' Helen pulled the bedroom curtains back rather more sharply than usual when she came in from the shower. 'And I want to know what was in that envelope you've hidden somewhere!'

'Oh, I *will* tell you darling,' he replied, at once anxious and trying to appease.

'And one more thing: I'm not letting anything get in the way of a holiday somewhere nice and warm. After all, psychiatrists retire a decade earlier than a lot of people, so my man of leisure should make the most of it.' Helen put her hands on his shoulders, smiled and kissed him.

'We'll have to see what we can do then,' he replied, looking into her eyes.

Helen went on getting ready. She had been working at the Squaremile Centre for the disabled for ten years, mostly as Manager of Sycamore House; now she wanted to go part-time so that they could be together more, with Max retired and both their girls at university. It was quiet each time Grace and Anna went away and it took some getting used to. Helen thought Max had earned a proper break too; at the same time, she feared that the fat folder might represent competition against a holiday, and was determined to find out what it was.

Max refused to be drawn; he was not about to embark on a lengthy explanation when Helen was going out.

'When you get back.'

'Owa. Can't you give me something to go on? Only if you're going to spend more time on that than on me, I think it's only fair you tell me about it.' She sat on the bed next to him, wrapped in her white robe, pretending to sulk. He took her hand and thought for a moment. She was looking at a bruise on her knee, while her freshly washed, neat black hair was slowly cascading over her face.

'Come back to bed.'

'I can't. I'm meeting Sally, remember?'

He watched Helen as she finished dressing. She looked at herself in the full-length mirror, turning and smoothing her clothes over her slim figure. He felt proud. He lay back on the bed, wanting to put off showering, wanting Helen. But he also knew he had to pick the right moment to ask for her help – and talk about Vee.

The next morning Helen seemed to be in a bad mood. She said she didn't want him to come with her to Howcester to get the groceries, thank you. The coating of snow was practically gone. She could manage, she said. So off she went, muttering and turning every small movement into a major event. Meanwhile, he sat in the living room, flicking through the holiday brochures Helen had picked up the day before, egged on, no doubt, by her friend Sally. He wondered why she was so huffy. Then the phone rang. It was Jim. Max remembered having scribbled his home number on the card he'd given him at the funeral. The young man had been to see his sister's grave, and wanted a quick chat.

'I've been meaning to ask you, Jim – where are your sister's ashes buried?'

'In St. Peter's, Howcester, with her father. Oh, and the inquest is on March 4th – but no doubt you'll get a letter.'

'Oh yes, thanks. By the way, Jim, I've decided to read the book. And I'm going to talk to Helen.' There was a loud clattering noise. 'Oh! that's the post. Hang on . . . ' There were a couple of cards. It explained Helen's mood. It was February 10th, their anniversary! 'Jim, I'm going to have to go now.'

'One last thing, Max: even though you and I have not worked together, I know your reputation. Social services will miss your contribution. Happy retirement!'

He'd better do something about this. They tended to ignore Valentine's Day because it was so close, but it meant doing *something*! She'd be back before long.

When Helen opened the front door with a large number of bags, Max came downstairs from the attic and pretended he'd forgotten the date to start with. He stalled. Next he tried to embrace her, but she had "all this shopping to put away". Then the florist's van turned up not a moment too soon, and he let her answer the door as if he couldn't be bothered.

'Oh, Max, you old devil! They're lovely. Come here!'

'Is Madame free zis evening?'

'Pourquoi?'

'Parce que I 'ave booked a tebell at ze Franch restaurant, Lisette's, for ett o'clock.'

'I might be.' She pretended to start sulking again, but couldn't keep it up. 'Would you like this?' She went over to the utility room and, reaching behind the door, pulled out the heavy country jacket, still in its polythene cover, that he had admired recently in a shop window. 'Try it on!'

'Oh, I'll try it on all right!' He chased her up the stairs and she shrieked in mock alarm.

They lay naked on the bed after making love. He looked at their reflection in the mirror opposite while playing about with their feet. It reminded him of how they used to be before the girls came along. Helen was staring at the ceiling; he noticed her cheek move.

'What are you smiling at, beautiful lady?'

'Oh, I was just thinking about when we first met.'

'On that bateau mouche on the Seine. Quite romantic, I s'pose.'

'I don't know if it was a bateau mouche, a vedette or a navette – I never really worked out the difference. But a boat of some sort, anyway. You were with your parents. You came over to ask me something, thinking I was French! When I didn't understand your best efforts – and I had you going there, didn't I, for a while! –' she laughed, 'you were embarrassed to discover that I was in fact from Edinburgh!'

He kissed her shoulder. 'It was a long way to go to find what was already at home.'

'Your parents; am I right in thinking that it was their first time abroad, ever?'

'You are. But I was worried that they were here in Howcester and I was so far away. I tried for two years to get a post down here, as you know, then when I did . . . It was as if I'd gone to Edinburgh just to meet you, pick you up and then take you away.

It was a shame my mum and dad weren't around long enough to make it to the wedding, but I shared yours.'

Helen laughed. 'Hey, Max. Isn't it nice to have time together, to talk?'

'Yes, darling.'

Helen was relieved to find the old Max again. For the past few months his sense of humour, important not only for his job, had been noticeably absent. The sex was better, too.

Propped up on one elbow, she recalled their time in Edinburgh.

'D'you remember how we used to meet up in that café near the Royal? You were like a teenager! Hadn't you had a girlfriend before me? I've been dying to ask you – I'm surprised I never got round to it. You were such a geek!' She smiled, that amazing smile. How could she upset anyone when she smiled like that? But for a moment he too pretended to sulk.

'Actually, I did have a girlfriend before you.' He smiled at her. 'But I behaved like that with you, I know, because you were a precious jewel. I was in awe; I couldn't believe you were mine.' As soon as he'd said this, he felt a pang: it was a wave of jealousy from Vee, watching, listening.

'Oh, Max! That's a lovely thing to say!' She went into her baby voice: 'But whatever you were, or are, like, I think you're dead sweet.' She dabbed him on the nose with her finger. 'The best hubby and the best daddy, ever.' Then she stretched, got up and pulled on her dressing gown, and resumed her usual voice. 'I'm cold!'

Max too stood up and began to get dressed. He decided that today would be the day he started reading Vee's book from the beginning.

Helen embraced her husband. 'I love having you all to myself. We don't need anyone else, do we? We've got two lovely daughters.' She smiled. 'And they all lived happily ever after,' she went on, musically, waving her index fingers as if conducting. Stopping abruptly, she added, 'Which reminds me, Mum wants to go to that concert after all, so –.'

'– Darling,' he interrupted, suddenly wanting to be serious. He still had to get her help.

'Yes? What's up?'

'Er . . . have you found out yet if you can go part-time?'

'You stopped the romantic mood to ask me *that* ?'

'Sorry, but there's something I want to – '.

' –Don't tell me you've got a mistress, some nubile young patient?'

'Oh no, nothing like that. I wouldn't have the time or the

energy, now would I, with all the demands *you* make in that department!'

They laughed, then kissed. He decided it was a good time.

'I need your help with something very important. And about that first girlfriend . . . '

5

Questions

Eventually, after reassurance that there had been nothing untoward – that is, recent – in their relationship, Helen was prepared to accept that Vee and Max had once been together, and she agreed to help him in whatever way she could. A few things now made sense to her about her husband's behaviour of late, and Max was contrite.

While neither of them knew precisely what Vee's demands might be, Helen was prepared for some kind of undercover work at Squaremile. At the end of their long discussion, which took the rest of that morning, they decided that they would *both* read *Doors Closing*.

'How about if I read one chapter, then pass it on to you?' Max sipped his coffee and Helen joined him in the conservatory.

'That sounds fine. Then, depending on what Vee has to say about Squaremile, we might be able to work out what to do. Her time there must feature in it. It must be one reason for her to write, don't you think? Oh, but Max, you'll never guess what . . . '

'What, my love?'

'They've told me I can't go part-time yet because they want "my experienced hand on the tiller" of Grove House, as they put it, in the not too distant future.'

'Why's that then?'

Helen gave a short, exasperated sigh. 'Sandra, the manager there at the moment, has somehow wangled a month's holiday.'

'A month? How come?'

'Lord alone knows. I'm afraid I don't have much time for

that woman.' Helen's Scots accent had become more notice-
able, as it often did when she was annoyed or stressed. 'She's
also tipped for promotion.' Helen slapped her thighs and
stood up. 'Don't get me started about Sandra.'

They had a quiet lunch together.

'I'm glad you've told me about your time with Vee,'
Helen said. 'I was worried about you.' She handed him an
apple.

'There might be other things I've forgotten to tell you, or
even that I didn't know, in connection with Vee. We'll find
out soon enough.' With that, Max headed off to the attic.

He had just picked up Vee's book when there was a knock
at the front door. Helen called him back down. He sighed
with frustration. To his surprise, it was Simon, pale.

'I'm in a bit of a state, Max.'

They went into the sitting room and Helen decided to
make some coffee.

'The truth is, Mark – that's my brother – has chucked us
out. Jackson's waiting in the car. Is there any chance we
might stay here for a while? I'll pay you some rent, of
course.' Simon gave a brief account, then fell silent. His
usual exuberance had evaporated. Max felt sorry for him.

Helen brought in the tray of coffee and Max put her in the
picture.

'Well,' she said, 'you can sleep in the girls' rooms until
they come back at the end of term, but then you'll have to
make other arrangements. Is that OK?'

Simon was grateful and fetched his son. Helen and Max
helped them in with their belongings. Jackson was fifteen
with a sullen expression, a spiky haircut and a t-shirt over
his sweater. When they saw the sound system, husband
and wife exchanged anxious glances. Helen went to change
the sheets; when he was sure Simon and Jackson were settled, Max went to his attic office and opened Vee's book at
last.

There was never going to be a "right" time for this and he
didn't want Simon to feel he was being watched either. He
thought about Vee, slipping over what might have been, and

turned to the first page. He lost himself in her story for a while.

Introduction

The story about Dad came a long time before the black wave that ripped my life apart. But I knew I had to write about it, how it all started, with the first bad thing in Granny's house.

I felt a sense of urgency; I had to write *now*, to avoid being stranded in hell by the next black wave; I couldn't afford to leave it too late, or I might not be able to do it. The problem is that I have no guarantee of complete recovery; when it comes, the black wave means I can't make sense of anything, or describe it to anyone, let alone remember where I'd got to in the story. And the treatment takes out memories.

After Dad, I kept writing, on and off for a few years in the end, and then realised I had started this book. I kept the diary separate; it was a place where I didn't have to be in control. Anyone can read the book. The diary, on the other hand, is for nobody but me.

I got over my homesickness at university – I was the first Gates to go there – by making new friends. There was one particular lecturer I admired, too, marked out by his incredible enthusiasm and knowledge of the subject. Mr Black could be sent into raptures by a passage from the French text we were reading; he would stride about the room, pausing only to scribble important points on the board, the sleeve of his gown flapping wildly. If we could not keep up and answer the questions he fired at us from time to time, he would get very annoyed. And then, for the whole of one term, he was simply not there. When he came back he looked pale and thin.

I noticed that my friend Debbie had also lost weight during this period but she didn't want to talk about it. On the first day of Mr Black's absence, she told me he was very ill and in hospital. She looked as if she hadn't slept, but she wouldn't say any more. I couldn't help wondering how she knew about him; I wasn't going to put pressure on her, however.

As for me, I was coping, but I confess that as the first year progressed, there were times, each lasting a few days, when I found it almost impossible to get out of bed. Everything was in monochrome. It was what I started to call the black wave, but as yet it was still not powerful enough to take me all the way to hell. Nevertheless, I knew that was its destination. I didn't feel I could tell Mum about this, so I went to talk to Debbie. I knocked on the open door of her room, one floor below me in the Hall of Residence. It was a typical study-bedroom. As I sat in the single armchair, Debbie tidied the books on her desk then sat on the bed.

'What's up, Vee?'

'Do you ever get days when you can't do anything and the world seems to be meaningless and grey?'

'Actually I do. I think I know what you're talking about. When it happened to me, I went to the doctor and he gave me those.' She pointed to a small bottle of pills next to the books. 'They have helped.'

I was in uncharted waters here. 'What are they?'

'Antidepressants.' There was a pause.

'But you don't need *tablets*, do you? I mean, I thought it was a case of, well, getting through it – pulling yourself together!'

'Oh, come on Vee, not that old chestnut! You know as well as I do that it's not as simple as that. Having mental health problems is not a sign of weakness!'

'Mental health – ? Yes, but it still feels like giving in!'

'Look, I'll lend you a book about depression and then you'll be able to form a proper opinion.'

'OK. Thanks.'

A moment later, she added, 'I know someone who is *manic* depressive.'

'What's that then?'

'It's when you have high moods as well as low. In other words, you can be full of enthusiasm and energy for a period

– more than normal – and you have lots of ideas crowding in. You might spend too much money, make extravagant plans, or even think you are someone with special powers. Mania can disrupt your life. But then you become the polar opposite, suicidally depressed. These moods can just come out of the blue.'

'I don't suppose you're going to tell me who it is that's got it?'

Debbie looked down. A secret smile was just visible between the curtains of her hair. 'No, but he's a lovely man.'

I have to admit I thought less of Debbie after that: she was weak, she had given in.

Even when someone was threatening to jump off the tallest building on campus, and I was in the crowd he attracted; even when I'd read Debbie's book and even when she wrote to me after we'd graduated to tell me Mr Black had committed suicide – not once did I think that my own problems were anything like this, or that other people knew about the black wave.

But then there was Aunt Mary . . . Mad people were all locked away though, weren't they? I reasoned, though, that I couldn't go on thinking Debbie was weak when I'd admired my lecturer so much. And I recognised, finally, that the student about to jump must have been tormented. Just around the corner was the connection I did not want to make.

I first met Aunt Mary at Granny's. Well, I didn't *meet* her exactly, but I probably got to know more about her than if I'd spoken to her.

Granny's telephone was ringing. When I was ten, it was kept for best with the piano in her front room. Jim and I were not allowed to play in there on our own. We didn't have a telephone or a piano at home, so Granny's rules were different. And she didn't want ink on the carpet.

'Hello. Mrs Wheeler speaking.'

That was the way you spoke to a telephone. When it rang,

it usually had bad news, so it was as well to be polite. Granny beckoned to Mum, who had to step over our toys to get to the doorway. Through the glass door I could see Mum's face change and Granny put her arm round her. Mum was upset. All this while Jim was making loud aerial bombing noises.

The news that we were to stay longer with Granny had been an exciting prospect. But even though we focused on visits to the sweet shop, with a whole shilling each, we were glad to hear the car. The Morris Minor engine stopped outside with a relieved rasp.

'Mummy, Mummy!' We rushed to the front door.

Good job she was back. We'd started to get bored and any day now we'd stop being good and let it show.

'Where have you been, Mummy?' asked Jim wearily. 'Have you brought us any presents?'

But Mum had brought us the first bad thing. I could tell that behind the control in her voice, something very bad was lurking. The words were like stilts wading precisely through deep, dark water. Jim was only six, too young to notice the significant looks which passed between the grown-ups; I never missed these looks, even though I knew I was meant to, because they came in little parcels of silence.

'Vee, Jim, come here and sit down.' She had to sound cold in order to keep talking, survive.

Even Jim was quiet then, sitting on the floor next to Granny's chair.

'Daddy won't be coming home.'

'Why not, Mummy? Where's he gone?' Jim frowned and fidgeted.

I could feel her suppressed sobs and wanted to cuddle her, make it stop. At the same time I knew that would be too dangerous for her.

'He's gone to . . . heaven.'

Jim was mystified.

'Now, you two,' said Granny, 'be good for your Mummy and go and pack up your things in the bedroom. Come on.' She was calm, but she meant it. She closed the bedroom door, then the hall door behind us while we listened. Then we heard a terrible, wounded animal scream and Jim tried to get out of the room. I stopped him, and he went and curled up on the bed instead, pretending not to cry.

This was the first bad thing.

A hot, still, summer day picture. Playing in the sand. Dad holding me round my middle, trying to teach me to swim in the sea. The colours are bright. Egg sandwiches before we left home early in the morning. Dad picking up fossils, telling me their names. Wild flower and bird names too.

I don't know how long it was after we were told, but one day I ran to my mother and sobbed into her soft dress.

'Hold the pen so the nib is at an angle – like this. Then do some up and down strokes like "n"s joined up.'

The headmaster went to each of us in turn, picking up our special pens and showing us how to slant the nib. There were about six of us in the Writers' Club, which met once a week in the front room of the headmaster's house next to the school. Most of the time we wrote stories, but today we were learning a new skill, while the fire cracked in the grate and the afternoon grew dark.

'That's good, Vee,' he said when he came back round to me. 'Now see if you can write your name like that, all of you.'

So "Vee Gates" was my first attempt at italic writing. I liked this school, but life so far had made sure I didn't get too attached to places. Before I knew it, I would probably have to move on again. This was my fourth primary school and I had got used to leaving people and places behind. Dad changed jobs quite often, so we had to keep moving house and living in all sorts of different towns. His last job had been on an oil rig in the North Sea. His brother, Uncle Ron, had been there for a while too. He was in one of the first gangs to be employed there when oil and gas were found; grown-ups were always talking about that. Mum had wanted to move up there nearer to Dad, as he seemed to be doing well.

But I was glad we hadn't moved, or I would have missed the Writers' Club.

My new uniform for the grammar school made a bit of a dent in the finances, but Mum battled on, finding work while I faced my new challenge. It was OK. As I said before, I had grown used to change, even if secretly I wanted things to stay the same, so I adapted without too much trouble. But I felt so much older now than Jim. And I became aware that I was much taller than the other girls in my class.

Uncle Ron had come round. He was two years younger than Dad, but Mum said they were like "peas in a pod". Mum was hidden from view by the back of the settee. She stood up. 'Uncle Ron's popped round to fix that leaking tap. Isn't he kind?'

Uncle Ron had become a frequent visitor recently, helping out in various ways around the house. He was an electrician by trade, but could turn his hand to more or less anything.

'When's dinner?' I asked.

'It won't be long. Could you get Jim in for me please?

'I'll be off now, Pam,' said Uncle Ron. 'You know where I am if you need me.'

One day when Uncle Ron wasn't there and Mum was dusting, I plucked up my courage. I thought Mum would be able to answer me now without getting upset, but I felt a surge of the black wave again all the same.

'Mummy?'

'Yes dear?'

'How did Daddy die?'

Mum looked at me. 'Come and sit down here and I'll tell you,' she said softly, patting the cushion next to her on the settee.

'You know he was on the rig?'

I nodded.

'Well, it was his job to climb up high. He was the derrickman, and that day his safety harness broke, so he fell down . . . ' She looked away. 'That's why I had to leave you at Granny's. I went to Oxford, where they'd brought him. D'you know, it's nearly a year ago . . . ' She stared straight ahead at the fireplace, then stood up quickly, marched across the room and picked up the framed photograph of Dad on the mantelpiece. Without a word, she placed it in the top drawer of the unit. Then she began dusting again and I knew she didn't want me there any more. So I slipped out of the room and went upstairs to start a new book. Beyond the sound of Jim playing cars, I heard Mum blow her nose. I felt sad that I was not enough for her, that she needed something I could not give.

These things are black drops, collecting, dripping into my mind. Each drop added itself to the total; a stream changed into a river, which would become an unnatural black tide.

'It's all women in this house!' said Jim, frustrated. 'God, I wish Dad was here.'

'Well he's not, so tough. And anyway, you don't remember him.' I was almost a teenager, practising a new spite.

'Yes I do!' His light grey eyes shone with indignation, but there was a touch of anxiety too.

Mum came out of the bathroom.

'If you want to see a film and have a picnic on Saturday, you'd better be good!'

Saturday was fun. When we got back home, Mum packed us off to bed. I thought it was unfair that I had to go to bed at the same time as Jim. I lay awake for a while, then realised that I couldn't hear anything downstairs. Mum and Uncle Ron had been talking and laughing and I hadn't heard the front door go to tell me he'd left. My curiosity got the better of me and I crept to the top of the stairs. Nothing, although lights were still on. Avoiding the creaky places, I went carefully down the stairs. If they heard me, I could say I wanted a drink of water.

Strange, muffled noises were coming from the living room. It sounded as if someone was being suffocated. Then there were sighs. Just then I tripped over the mat in the hall.

There was a gasp and Mum's head appeared above the back of the settee. 'Vee! What're you doing out of bed?'

'I . . . came down to see if . . . I mean, for some water. Are you alright?'

'Yes, fine. Uncle Ron was just leaving, weren't you?'

I couldn't see or hear him, but I worked it out.

'Back to bed, Vee.'

The next day I managed to talk to Mum, while she was putting some washing out.

'Mum, do you love Uncle Ron?'

'He's been a good friend.' She would not be drawn.

I had uncovered a new dimension to my mother. Until now, I had not seen her as attractive, or as a woman for that matter. Nor had it occurred to me before that day that Uncle Ron's visits had any other purpose apart from helping out.

'Are you going to marry him?'

Mum moved the basket along and paused before picking up a shirt. 'I don't know. He hasn't asked me yet.'

'If you do get married, do we have to call him Dad?'

'No, darling.'

When Uncle Ron moved in with us six months later, I realised that if they did marry, at least we wouldn't have to change our name.

Grandpa had sold the butcher's business at the back of his childhood home, The Elms, and the house was going to rack and ruin; just after my fourteenth birthday, Mum decided that the time had come to turn the place out. I was able to help her and Granny as we were now in the summer holidays.

'This is what the house used to look like,' Mum said, picking out a black and white photograph from the box Uncle Ron had brought down from the loft. I studied the picture.

'And here's my dad, Grandpa, when he was about four, with his mother – your great-grandmother.' The young

woman wore Edwardian dress which showed off her slim
waist and both she and Grandpa stared seriously at the
camera. I thought how much Jim looked like this boy in a
sailor suit. 'And here are the Wheelers, on chairs, with their
servants sitting on the lawn; see their aprons and caps?'

Grass was just the same and clouds were just the same,
and these people once breathed just like us. I looked along
the row of unsmiling Wheelers, recognising here and there
some facial features.

'So tell me who they all are, Mum.'

'There's James, your great grandfather, Sarah you've just
seen with Grandpa – here he's about ten – and that's Aunt
Mary.'

'Who was she?'

'She was Grandpa's older sister.'

'I didn't know he had a sister! What happened to her? Is
she still alive?'

'No, she died a long time ago.'

'But he's never said anything about her!'

'Oh, well. People don't always say everything about
themselves. And anyway, she had a difficult life.'

'What do you mean?'

Mum pulled her lips tight. This expression meant she
didn't want to tell you something. 'I expect you'll find out
one day.'

'But I want to know now!' I exclaimed.

Over the next few days I tried several times to find out
about Aunt Mary, but as each effort was met with a change
of subject or an attempt to divert my attention, I gave up in
the end. Adults always got their way, especially when they
were balancing on the edge of a bad thing.

Granny, Mum and I spent three or four days sorting
things out at The Elms, while Jim had time with Uncle Ron,
who had taken a week off. We found clothes, books, letters,
postcards strewn about, ornaments, vases and all kinds of
remnants of people's lives, coated in dust and grit. Mum told
me that when she first went there, she'd found the skeleton
of a cat in a drawer: Grandpa's mother was stone deaf. Most

of the windows were broken, and weeds were beginning to colonise the downstairs rooms, among the remains of carpets. I remember sitting on a patch of bare floor, studying the old books with their elaborate covers, tissue paper and engravings, determined not to move from that spot when I was alone in case I came across another skeleton.

Among other things, Mum brought some of the clothes home with us on the first day. She held up one item, a kind of smock, with an open back which tied at the neck. I could tell that she wished she hadn't. When I insisted on knowing what it was, Mum had to say that it was the sort of thing Aunt Mary might have worn when they "took her away". I didn't understand what this expression meant, but all Mum would say was that I'd find out one day, and that I wasn't to ask any more questions.

That night I dreamt about Aunt Mary. She was being led away like a dog on a lead, on all fours, her tongue too far out and her white eyes rolling. She was panting and the white eyes just kept on rolling in their sockets. I was terrified, but it was babyish to call for Mum. But when this dream came three nights in a row, I knew I had to do something about Aunt Mary. I decided to shut her away behind a white door in my head. The door had to be secure. It was set in a white-washed brick wall, the front of a building which was not visible. This was the second bad thing, even though I could not imagine what Aunt Mary could do to me. Unfortunately, though I hardly ever called it to mind deliberately, the white door had come into being and was now a feature in my private mental landscape. I thought I knew what it concealed.

6

Schools

I was better off concentrating on schoolwork. We stayed put in Howcester for the next few years, long enough for me to take my 'A' levels.

I met all kinds of girls, jealous ones, bullies, quiet kind ones, girls whose writing you wanted to copy, girls whose new things you envied, girls you just couldn't stand, but there seemed to be three main categories in all this: the swots, most of whom wore glasses, the quiet drippy ones, some of whom had specs and the fashion squad, none of whom wore glasses, and wouldn't have worn them on principle even if they'd needed to. Even though I didn't misbehave, and I felt guilty and sorry for the poor student teacher, trying so hard at the front of our class, I wasn't sure which category I fitted into until I was sixteen, just before 'O' levels, when my eyes decided they belonged to a swot.

I was fed up with all the changes I'd been going through and to have swotness added to the list was the last straw. Officially a woman for a couple of years now, I still wanted to play football with the boys. Mum and Ron put a stop to that. I didn't think much of this woman business – it spoilt everything. We learned about all sorts of embarrassing things in biology too; the teacher went into much more detail than Mum.

While all around me girls were experimenting with make-up and going out with boys, I was still expected to get on with my work as I had always done. Mum said there would be plenty of time for "All That" later, although I did go to a few parties and listen to some pop music. But my glasses went before me, proclaiming my swotness, and I found it difficult to make friends. At school there were girls, mostly members of the fashion squad, who already had a sense of their own identity and a freedom in their behaviour which was alien to me; it enabled them to get away with almost anything without any very severe punishment. I felt sure that if *I* had done those things, all hell would have broken loose, especially if Mum were to find out. We'd had teenage rows at home of course, especially of the door-slamming variety, with my parting shot to Ron, "You're not my dad!"

By the time I reached the Sixth Form though, most of the colourful characters and the quiet drips had left. Those who remained from these groups seemed to have realised something serious: they had grown up. And now, of course, my glasses were a kind of badge. Aunt Mary was still there, but I had pushed some big boxes full of books against the white door. It was a very ordinary adolescence, but the black drops were still dripping, out of sight.

I had all the usual childhood ailments, and Mum looked after me, but Ron always seemed to think I was doing it for attention, so that over time, being ill and feeling guilty became inseparable in my mind. It had to be my fault; I was letting everyone down. And I didn't see any need to discuss this mindset because I thought everybody's household worked the same way. Likewise, I had accepted the presence of Aunt Mary as part of ordinary life. Not something you talked about every day, but there all the same.

But I was not just a swot in the Sixth Form: I had to get everything right. Because to get things wrong was to invite the black wave. While I might have believed I was in a position of strength, in fact it was simple arrogance, which is the armour of the insecure. My disdain spread to people who had anything wrong with them, like my grandparents who had let themselves get old and deaf. I found it hard to conceal my impatience. But the worst offenders were those who showed any sign of being "mental". Nothing was going to go wrong for me: I was in control. I knew exactly how the black wave could come, where Aunt Mary and the door were, and how to limit their influence. I had absolute faith in a state of eternal health, along with what I considered intellectual superiority – and oh yes, I sealed my contemptuous perfectionism with a determination never to get old. I wasn't weak!

I tried to read one of the course books on the train south to uni, but it was difficult. Fields passed and trees rushed by and I thought about Aunt Mary. I had really wanted to ask Granny about her, but I never seemed to find the right time.

Why had she been "taken away"? Did it happen more than once? I recalled the old dream of her as a dog on a lead. Secretly I knew the answer, but it was hard to admit to having a relative who must have been mentally ill. I checked the white door: it was still closed, the boxes of books were still there and it was partially obscured by ivy.

My routine was totally different now and I had very little money, but much more freedom than at school; it was up to each of us to structure our day. This took some getting used to, as did sharing a kitchen and bathroom with complete strangers.

After graduating and getting a PGCE, I soon discovered that to teach was not simply to convey knowledge to a rapt audience. It was hard work. I could see so many different personalities and needs in each class. But I was still naïve enough to believe that my love of French would enable me to impart my knowledge without any trouble, a belief that was soon to be utterly destroyed.

My first full-time job was in a comprehensive in the Midlands. The buildings were of the plain 1960s variety. In some places the roof leaked, and the paint was peeling, but the staff worked on regardless. Most were disillusioned, punch-drunk and demoralised, inured to the dismal round of coping with adolescent minutiae, doing their best in spite of everything, day in, day out. Cynicism, it seemed, was all that kept them going. They seemed to have forgotten how to live in any other way.

I walked into a classroom one day to find two boys fighting. The rest of the class, a bunch of streetwise fourteen-year-olds, were cheering and egging them on. I went to the front and shouted.

'Kevin and Sean, break it up! Now! Everybody sit down. Come on! Quiet! Sit down, Tracy.

'Miss, Miss!' Tracy shouted from the back. 'He's doin' sumfink disgustin'!'

I didn't know what to do. I still did not understand why discipline was not automatic.

'Eeurrh! Two or three boys stood up. 'I'm not sittin' next to him, Miss!' said Jason. 'He's filfy!'

'Miss! Sean's bleedin.' Can I go to Mrs Jones wiv 'im?'

'Oh, alright.'

'Pwaar! Who's farted?' came another voice, followed by a peal of laughter. 'Can I open the window, Miss?'

Meanwhile I was trying to write something on the board, which was being pelted with bits of chewed-up paper meant for the back of my head. I turned round quickly and saw two boys hide something.

'Miss?'

'Yes, Sharon?'

'Why do we 'ave to learn French. It's borin.' We'll never go to France, anyway. Who wants to? Bloody frogs!'

This comment set off more laughter as well as croaking noises. I couldn't give Sharon an honest answer, because in the end, Set 3 were never going to be able to get anywhere with their French. The idealism of teaching theorists would soon evaporate in this room. The truth was, I could see the children's point of view, a fact which naturally undermined me. They weren't there from choice, and they might have had problems at home, something which never crossed my mind at the time. Only dimly aware of it, I was digging a hole for myself with the class looking on. I wanted to keep up the appearance of being strong in adversity, so I ignored what my instincts told me. Uncle Ron had taught me to be tough, not to give in, not to complain. But my attempts to get past the issue of discipline and into the safer territory of actual teaching only served to make me more and more weary. The problem would not go away. Things rapidly reached the stage where I could not climb out of the hole. The black wave was up, ready to carry me to hell.

My private insecurity was now on public display. Only in teaching do you stand exposed in this way, and only children are capable of rubbing away at your very soul until it dawns on you that all is lost. Then there is the heart-stopping, instant silence which tells you that another teacher has entered the room, an especially vivid reminder of your shortcomings if the teacher is there because your class was disturbing the one next door. The children searched in vain for someone in me who would stand up to them. I could feel the black wave twisting, threatening to burst through. I stayed at home for a couple of days, feeling empty and not knowing what I should do.

'You're depressed,' said Wendy, a fellow teacher who found me in bed. 'Go and see the doctor.'

One of my flatmates had let her in; the school was concerned at my absence. But the doctor was no help at all, telling me to go away and sort out my problems. She must have thought I was weak. I was. I was useless. Aunt Mary . . . The padlock was broken, the boxes had been moved.

When I failed my probationary year it should have come as no great surprise. But it was the first time I had ever tasted failure. I had always taken it for granted that I would succeed in whatever I did, if not from ability then out of determination, toughness. Something died in me that day. I discovered that getting things right all the time was impossible. I was, after all, a weak person. To my shame I packed up and travelled back to Howcester to stay with Mum. At least she and Ron were there for me.

'So what are you going to do next?' Mum asked one morning. 'Do you want to retrain?'

'No. I want to teach.'

'But how d'you plan on doing that?' She began the washing-up.

'I can apply to independent schools. They might give me

another chance to prove I can do it.' I picked up the tea towel.

'Oh, Vee! I forgot to tell you! You know your old grammar school?'

'Yes?'

'Well, they've moved everyone out to another site. They've had to knock the old place down. Something to do with concrete fatigue . . . '

I had spent seven years at that school, but I didn't get attached to places, did I? So what was this uncomfortable feeling?

It was getting late, so Max closed the folder. With Simon and Jackson living in their house though, it was difficult to relax. Max did feel sorry for them, but he hoped they would soon find somewhere else. Helen was fed up. After reading these first pages, Max wrote:-

"It is clear that Vee's childhood was unremarkable, apart from the death of her father. She had been loved, but the spectre of Aunt Mary haunts her." Then he realised that this Uncle Ron must have been the tall gentleman with Mrs Gates he'd seen at the funeral.

He went on: "Despite the difficulties she experiences in her early career, Vee evinces the determination she will need as her life moves on through light and shade. *I* haven't appeared in the story yet, and my anxiety is edging up a bit. But I know from the way things are going that Vee is about to move to Lexby, so no doubt I will be in it soon. I can't recall what it was like not to know Helen, though. She now has Vee's first pages. Incidentally, Helen has read nothing of what *I've* written; she wanted to, but I said I would only let her after we've read Vee's book.

"The big question of action remains. I might be committing myself to much more in the way of personal involvement, in ways I have not yet considered. Meanwhile I will read on, to escape domestic chaos as much as anything else – Simon knows what I'm doing and has left me to it. Vee's story is made of the kinds of things you get to know about someone when you are close to them for long enough. While she did not have that opportunity with me, I can still feel her watching, somewhere near".

7

A Mind for Change

It was hard to get to sleep that night because Simon's son Jackson had some friends round who didn't leave until midnight and played loud music. Helen and Max had forgotten just how noisy teenagers could be. They asked the boys to turn it down when they went to bed at eleven, but after a hollow apology Max heard sniggering from the boys and it wasn't long before the music was as loud as before. Simon was nowhere to be found. Max would not have been surprised if Jackson's behaviour had contributed significantly to their eviction by Simon's brother.

Helen and Max were forced to lie awake until the boys decided to pack up. Max heard Simon come back at around 2 a.m. Then there was the bathroom. Not only a queue in the mornings but scum round the bath. And then Helen found a half bottle of vodka in the cupboard under the washbasin.

As he sat wearily in his attic office, about to read Vee's next chapter, the light changed and Max was back in the pitch black lecture theatre. Darkness, apart from the spotlight on him and the irregular lace effect of the light at the top of their heads. When a student speaks, his or her face is illuminated as if by a torch. Eerie though the setting may be, Max proceeds as if nothing unusual were happening.

"Can anybody give me a definition of good mental health?" There is silence. Then Mr Phillips's face appears as he says:

"It means having your life in balance, keeping interested in things, not doing anything to excess – and getting enough rest." The torch clicks off.

"Fine, those are certainly aspects of it, but to my knowledge, nobody has ever summed it up succinctly. We have precise tools for diagnosing illness, and we can usually tell when somebody is unwell, but more often than not, we have to fall back on 'the absence of illness' as our unspoken definition, despite what this could mean. The WHO's definition of health in general includes the words: 'a state of complete well-being', but that doesn't help really, does it? And how would you define that other old chestnut, 'normal'?"

"That's a bit easier, sir," says Mr Jones, his features animated in the light, "because it has a social context." Click.

"Explain."

"Well, every society has rules and behaviour which are considered 'normal', even though one society's normal might be another's weird."

There is a short burst of laughter in the dark from the four tiers of young men and women, all in darkness.

"That's good enough for now, but it's important to bear in mind that, whatever the social context, the differences between well/unwell, normal/abnormal, are not necessarily clear-cut – or even constant. So. Our next topic: severe depression. Symptoms can be quite unmistakeable. What does psychomotor retardation mean, Mr Phillips?"

"It means, sir, that the patient is slow physically, so they have difficulty walking, eating, etc." His torch goes out.

"Right. Their thought processes are slow, too. In fact if the depression is extreme, they can go into stupor – I'm not going to talk about that right now – but in that state, they must be kept under observation."

The face of a young woman appears in the dark: "Would ECT be the treatment of choice for someone as depressed as this?"

"It depends on the individual circumstances, but I have seen patients who have undergone a remarkable recovery with ECT. The argument against it relies mainly on the fact that we don't know how it works. But the same could be said of many of the medications we prescribe."

The students murmur. Then Mr Flint speaks, his round face like a moon: "What do you think about the stigma attached to mental illness?" Click.

"If people lost their jobs every time they had a cold, they would soon protest. But that's what it can be like for people with a mental illness. When you think that one in four people at any given time are in the throes of a mental illness, you can see how illogical stigma is – it is born of fear and ignorance."

The darkness lifted and he was back in the attic. Fiery red and orange lines – that's what he used to draw on the board in his talks to represent failure, prejudice and discrimination – they were the threat.

He wrote:-

"Because of what we the onlookers might be feeling, it is easy to miss the fear – drawn as a ragged black blob underneath the rearing colours – which a patient experiences: I knew that Vee was terrified when she began to relapse. Mental illness, the glass box round all my drawings, is not seen as a struggle in the same sense as, perhaps, a battle against cancer.

"Becoming ill is all about losing control, which is not the same as giving in. Vee never gave in, but she feared losing control: her black wave. In terms of hostile environments, however, teaching was lower down the scale than what was to come. Oh yes, it was going to get worse for Vee.

"Then there was guilt. Guilt was an empty sphere in the corner of this picture, which could grow and fill like a balloon, but filling with lead, not air. And what about the fear of change, represented by a jagged blue line along the bottom? Vee had had plenty of change in her life, so she wasn't afraid of that in itself. But at Squaremile, she was to discover that change is not always for the better. I know this from what Bella has told me. And another thing: even if it is welcomed, change entails stepping into the unknown.

"Finally, as a result of her experiences at Squaremile, Vee's belief that you were not worthy of love unless you had never failed at anything, academic or emotional, seemed to be confirmed. So there is the 'R' stamp in the middle, obliterating much of the drawing. Reject".

Vee had been afraid of becoming ill, afraid of failure and afraid of love, each a part of losing control in some sense. But at the same time, ironically, she displayed great persistence. Someone else who knew the meaning of persistence was his darling Helen.

As he glanced along his bookshelf and saw her photo, he remembered Edinburgh. The gusty wind reminded him of the city too. Helen was doing her nurse's training, he was a brand new consultant, he'd only been there about six months, and they used to meet in a busy café. From the start, from their first encounter in Paris, he'd felt the rightness of it. His time in Lexby with Vee faded into the background, his love for her became dormant as Helen moved into the foreground.

Any number of things might have prevented that first meeting, and yet here she was, Helen, wanting to be with him, sitting opposite him by the window. She was talking to him, pointing things out in the street, but he couldn't hear what she was saying because he was overwhelmed by the wonderful fact of her presence, her amazing eyes, her beautiful, expressive hands . . .

"Max, are you OK? Only you didn't answer my question."

"Sorry . . . er, what did you say?"

"What time have you got to be back at the Royal?"

"Oh – now!" he stood up and put some money on the table.

"Call me!" She smiled to herself as he headed out towards a sunlit Morningside.

While Max was working at the Royal Edinburgh Hospital, Helen made their first few weeks together an adventure. As she had been born and brought up in the city, she was able to show him round. Edinburgh is amazing, full of contrasts, not least where the weather is concerned. Of course they saw all the tourist sites and places of interest in the area: the castle, various monuments and several museums for example; Max had particularly enjoyed the National. They walked their legs off.

Max appreciated the fact that as well as knowing the cultural highlights, Helen knew all the right restaurants and cafés to go in, when they were too shattered to walk any further. They were both free at the weekend and spent most of the time together. Max remembered those Sunday mornings in her flat, in bed by her side one minute, then smelling the toast the next, and hearing her sing in the kitchen. He had the wonderful, comfortable feeling that he could say anything to Helen and she would understand. He could tell she was totally at ease as well. This was going to work.

Coming back to the present in Howcester, he steeled himself to read the next chapters: Lexby was imminent. Once again, he had to try to be objective, a difficult task when he remembered the special party. Although aware that Vee's account was allowing him a greater insight than usual into another's thoughts, Max also had to bear in mind his main reason for reading the book: to find out what she wanted him to do.

Castlebrough School for girls, in Lexby on the south coast, was in fact a row of five imposing houses dating from the early 1900s. They had been converted in the '50s and were linked at the back by a covered way. The sound of deep gravel in the parking area dignified the arrival of my taxi.

'Miss Gates?'

'Yes.'

'Do come in. I'm matron. If you wouldn't mind waiting in here, Miss Henshaw will be with you in a moment.' She smiled graciously and I sat in a corner of a large room, my stomach fizzing with nerves.

Miss Henshaw, the headmistress, was a short, round, pink woman of about fifty. She had a slight Irish accent. After my interview, in the few anxious minutes alone in that room with the high white ceiling, I knew I would have to say something: when Miss Henshaw reappeared, I admitted that I'd failed my probation. I could not look at her and the seconds passed. Her tone of voice did not alter, however.

'I would like to offer you the post of French teacher,' she said. 'I'll see you in September. And thank you for your honesty.'

While my first thought was that Miss Henshaw must have been desperate to fill the post, the next moment I felt optimistic. Having passed my driving test in Howcester, the first thing I did was buy a car.

A few years would pass with no hint of trouble, no sign of the black wave, making me think the dream of Aunt Mary was just that, a dream, an ineffectual force.

8

Affairs at Lexby

The staffroom was full of sunlight the first time I went in; the enormous windows faced south east.

'You'll be in charge of the French teaching,' my new head of department told me. Miss Gibson was tall and thin and had a strange laugh, which seemed to require a lot of effort. She was responsible for the German teaching.

'So – right through to 'A' level?'

'Yes. The classes here are small, much smaller that I expect you've taught before, so you'll get to know the girls quite quickly. I've been here ten years and I love it.' She gave one of her laughs, which resembled deep-seated panting. 'And there's very little in the way of serious disruptive behaviour. After all, their parents are paying, and they'd soon hear if anything happened. The girls come from all over the world, you know.'

I realised I was the youngest teacher there. And at last I could now do what I'd always wanted to do: enjoy my work. Marking in the evenings was nowhere near as daunting as before, and I could give individual attention more easily.

On the subject of individual attention, the brand new computer room was opposite the staffroom in House 1: I was to spend some time in there, though not necessarily occupied with computing. Tony taught IT, when it had just emerged from maths as a separate subject. We found we were attracted to each other. On the last day before half-term, when as usual there was sherry in the staffroom, Tony went across the way to pack up his things. I teased, flirted. The sherry was strong.

'You keep on like that and I'll be round your flat.'

I draped myself up the doorframe when the coast was clear. 'Can if you want.' The sexual tension between us about to find release, I drove home and waited, nervous but excited by the secrecy. I had only had one boyfriend up to then.

I lived on the top floor of a forties semi, near the railway line. It belonged to one of the other teachers and I paid a low rent because one room was full of his stuff. All the bedroom furniture was in dark wood and there was a flimsy camp bed in the corner. Everything seemed to be tidy today. But now here was Tony's car. My heart jumped and I went down to let him in. He was married, so we had to be discreet, but right now discretion was the last thing on our minds. The kissing was powerful, our clothes went everywhere. It was sheer lust and it felt good, perhaps because of the guilt.

Then one day Miss Henshaw came into the computer room and we had to put our hands away. 'Ah, Miss Gates. I didn't know you were interested in computers!'

I knew I looked guilty. 'I . . . I'm having lessons,' I managed.

'I see. How's she doing, Mr Brown?'

'Oh,' Tony gave a nervous laugh. 'Shaping up nicely!'

This unfortunate expression didn't help at all; Miss Henshaw looked at each of us in turn, raised her eyebrows, nodded sagely and walked out. I sighed. I suppose she could hardly say, "Keep it up!" could she?

Tony and I met regularly for a while at my flat, but with Christmas coming, he would be needed more at home. And my downstairs neighbours complained to my landlord about the bedroom noises. A camp bed on bare boards. Rather embarrassing to recall.

But worse was to come.

'I heard of two teachers once,' began Mrs Selby, science, as she addressed the group round the staffroom table one lunchtime. 'They used to meet once a week – oh, yes, and at the end of term, after the sherry.'

Luckily I had my back to them, but I sensed that the others were smiling as they got the message. My skin tingled.

'He was married, but his car was seen outside her flat.'

I dared not try to catch Tony's eye. It would have meant turning my head and it was not difficult to imagine that I was being watched.

'They thought nobody knew, but you could tell which day of the week it was – at least, so I'm told.'

When the time came for afternoon lessons, I found it hard to know where to look and wanted to escape from the staffroom as unobtrusively as possible. But I nearly knocked over the Christmas tree in the foyer. Nowadays I would probably have smiled at Mrs Selby as if I hadn't recognised myself.

Ben's motorbike pulled up. Tony and I were in the bedroom. I knew Ben fancied me, but I wasn't expecting him. I panicked, threw on my dressing gown, Tony grabbed his clothes and fled into the bathroom. 'Let him in, Vee! Tell him you were just about to have a bath!'

'But he'll see your car!'

'Yes, and you can say I've only just turned up. Something needed fixing or something. Go!' He slammed his feet into his shoes.

But I couldn't carry it off. Ben went home. Tony was furious. When we started the new term in January, I knew that Ben had worked it out. They spoke to each other but not to me: I was the scarlet woman. There was not going to be any more hanky panky on the camp bed: shame is a big obstacle to passion.

I had never fallen in love. I'd had lustful flings, but that was about it. I couldn't really see a future with the expected husband and children. That world was closed to me and I did not deserve to enter it. Marriage signified a higher level of being, of acceptance in society than I could ever hope to attain: if you failed or you weren't tough, you were unworthy of love. I just had to accept this fundamental truth. I was simply inferior. Even though the wound from my first job had healed enough for me to succeed at Castlebrough, there was a scar. My guilt over the affair with Tony made things worse in the end. And keeping in touch with Mum, Ron and Jim was difficult as I was not on the phone in my flat. I was lonely. But as I said, not once did the black wave threaten. The whole thing seemed to have gone for good.

Joan Gibson hardly ever interfered with what I was doing in the classroom; if she did have something to say, it would always be with her apologetic, panting laugh. Because I felt strong in this environment, where I had control, it was easier for me to deal with any minor misbehaviour. One day in my first term, I picked up my books and headed along the covered way to House 3. I know you're not supposed to have favourites as a teacher, but everyone does. You just have to be careful.

'I think you'll find they're in room 9,' a colleague whispered to me in the corridor as I searched for 2H, normally in room 4. She smiled knowingly and patted me on the arm. As I got nearer to room 9, I heard "ssshh! ssshh!" There was silence as I walked in.

'Bonjour la classe!'

Their reply was punctuated by giggles and snorts of suppressed laughter. 'Bon . . . jour, Mademoi . . . selle!'

I turned to the board. 'Now copy this down in your rough books: "I must stay in the right classroom so that my teacher knows where I am."' I gave them a few moments, then when heads started to come up, I added: 'And . . . translate it into French.' Of course I knew that they were only having a bit of harmless fun, but I still had to have the last word.

'Miss?' Caroline had her hand up.

'Yes, Caroline?'

'Miss, it's . . . it's too hard.' There was a murmur of agreement.

'Well now, I thought that perhaps being in a fifth form classroom might make it easier. Ah, yes. It needs a subjunctive. Right, will you all, quietly, go back to room 4.' I allowed them to see a slight smile. We understood each other.

They soon turned into 3H, then 4H, and they started their 'O' Level work, blossoming into young women. Once the summer exams were over, all the classes relaxed and some even had their lessons in the school grounds under the magnificent spread of the old trees, or were allowed to use the pool more often. These slow and lovely years almost lulled me into forgetting about change.

It was rare for Miss Henshaw to come into the staffroom. One lunchtime I saw Tony holding the door open for her. We all fell silent. She looked round the room and invited us to sit down if we could. She looked at her watch, then began:

'I have something very important to tell you. As I expect you know, the school is suffering from falling rolls.'

Somebody coughed. Someone else whispered to a friend.

'It has been decided therefore,' she went on, 'that Castlebrough will amalgamate with Stoneleigh College down the road. This will take effect from January next year, and we will be moving into the buildings you have no doubt seen under construction next to the College. The new school will be called Stonecastle. Let us hope it will last as long as its name suggests.' There were anxious murmurs. 'If any of you wish to discuss your options, come and see me.' With that, she swept out of the staffroom.

'You know what this means, don't you?' exclaimed Ben. 'It'll be *all* the teachers competing for *half* the jobs!'

'Thank you *so* much for that, Ben. What it is to be good at maths!' Mr Gray, history, slammed down a pile of books and stomped out of the room.

The anxiety spreading like fire around the room left me untouched, because it had only taken me a matter of seconds to decide that I would leave. For one thing, I knew it would not be difficult for me to find another job now and for another, I had learned not to get too attached to places, hadn't I? I kept a cool head and let Miss Henshaw know what I was planning. I must admit, though, that the tension in the staffroom was unbearable at times. While I did feel sorry for those nearing the end of their careers in this quiet backwater, I took no part in any more staffroom business, focusing on my lessons and my interviews.

Interviews. The travelling and keeping smart is bad

enough, but the worst part is always waiting for the result, especially if you're not told at the time. Every time the phone rang I felt a fizz of nerves. Then it came. Ben handed me the receiver. A deep male voice was at the other end:

'Miss Gates? Ah, it's the headmaster of Arnold College, West Pluting here. I am pleased to tell you that we would like to offer you the post of French teacher. I shall of course be writing to confirm this. Do you accept?'

'Yes. Thank you.'

'In that case, we look forward to your joining us in September.'

I needed to keep a lid on my excitement for the time being, however. Quite apart from the fact that it would not have been very tactful to start celebrating at work, there was something I had to do which was not going to be easy.

When 4H had settled, I gave them some written work. As I walked round the desks, the dark floorboards creaked like an old ship and I thought about what I would say. For the first time at Castlebrough, I realised, I felt the presence of the black wave. It was nearly time; I asked them to close their books.

'Girls, there's . . . I've got something to tell you. At the end of term, on Thursday, I shall be leaving.'

Utter silence. I found it hard to look at them. Then one girl flung herself forward on her desk and wailed, 'Now I *will* fail my French 'O' Level!' The bell sounded and they filed out with scarcely a sound, avoiding my gaze: collectively they knew that to appear hostile was the easiest option. When they had gone, I cleaned the board, then sat at the front for a moment, feeling cold on a warm day.

9

Party and Parting

The view from Diane's garden was breathtaking. The sun was setting, flame red, into the sea, bathing the guests and the marquee in an exotic glow and making the unlit side of people's bodies look blue, as if they were part of an impressionist painting. Diane taught PE at Castlebrough. Her fiancé, Jeff, sold expensive cars for a living and had bought the grand Victorian house for them six months earlier. I watched them now as they set about lighting torches around the garden, defining it in the dusk.

The engagement party was getting underway – an excellent end to the term. About forty people, most of them unknown to me, were here to celebrate. Every so often a cheer would go up above the general noise with the pop of another champagne cork. I was wearing contact lenses nowadays and my favourite smart outfit tonight, though I soon ditched the heels because of the grass.

Diane came towards me, smiling, her eyes and necklace catching the flickering light. She was wearing a long, sleeveless cream dress and her hair was up.

'You look lovely,' I said. "Lady in Red" was playing.

'So do you. Have you met Jeff?'

He joined her and she put her arm round him.

'You must be Vee.' He smiled. 'Sad the old school's going, isn't it?'

'Yes, but we have to move on sometimes, don't we?' I replied.

Diane now linked her arm in mine. 'Excuse us, Jeff, but there's someone over there who's itching to meet you, Vee!' She steered me towards a small group who'd just opened another bottle. 'Hi Steve, nice to see you; this is Vee. Vee this is Mark, and his wife Louise. And Max, this is Vee. Vee, meet Max Greenwood.'

'Hello,' said Max. 'Shall we go over there and sit down a minute? Oh – would you like some champagne?'

'Yes please.'

His extraordinary blue eyes spoke of a kindness and intelligence which startled me. Max brought me a glass and we sat by a small table, facing out to sea. The water was dark now and peaceful; only the wavelets breaking on the shore were visible by the streetlamp on the promenade below us.

'So. I teach French. What do you do?'

'I'm a doctor,' said Max. He smiled, his eyes shining in the torchlight. With the sunset, the glow on the faces had shifted from coral to amber yellow. 'Vee. Is that short for anything?'

'Yes. Victoria, but that's what my mother used to call me when –'

'– you did something wrong. I know. I can still hear it: *"Maxwell!"*' We laughed.

'So where do you do your doctoring?' I asked, feeling the champagne.

'At the hospital here in Lexby. Well, for the moment.' We looked in the direction of the latest cheer, but quickly returned to exploring each other's face again.

'I've just been offered –' We said this together, then laughed again.

'You go first!'

'OK. I'm off to a new job down in West Pluting. D'you know it at all?'

'No, not really,' he replied. 'Teaching French again?'

'Yes. Your turn.' I couldn't suppress a giggle.

'My new job's in Edinburgh; it'll be my first consultant's post.'

I felt a thread of disappointment which I couldn't quite explain. 'Wow! In what field?'

'Psychiatry.' There was a pause. Max smiled again. 'Does that put you off?'

'Not at all. When do you start?'

'Next month. Are you looking forward to your new job –
in September, I take it?'

'Yes. It looks like a challenge. It's a much bigger school.'

Max poured some more champagne, then we looked at
each other again for a moment, this time with a smile which
refused to fade. Strangely, I felt no embarrassment, no need
to look away. He was a few years older than me, his dark
hair thinning slightly at the front. Then he went to get us
some food. I noticed Diane looking at me from across the
garden. She had CDs of all the 'eighties hits.

'So how come you know Diane, then?' I asked when he
got back.

'It's not Diane I know but Jeff. We were at Oxford together
– a few years ago now, of course. Then I came here and
wanted to buy a car and who should I meet but Jeff.' Max
raised his glass to Jeff, who noticed and came over to join us
with Diane for a short while, bringing up a couple more
chairs, those lovely white metal ones which look like frozen
lace.

'Vee,' said Diane, turning her head conspiratorially to one
side for a moment and beckoning me to do the same. 'You
seem to be getting on well with Max. We must keep in touch.
Ring me when you start your new job – or if you don't!' She
had a mischievous glint in her eye as she smiled and flapped
her hand, pretending not to want to know any more and
moving on to another group.

I watched Max, deep in conversation with Jeff. Why did I
have to meet him right now, when our lives were going in
completely different directions? I glanced at the sea and
wondered how anyone ever finds stability. How do people
ever *feel* good enough to spend their lives with someone
else? Come to think of it, how does the chance come along
which allows them to do that? I spent the rest of the evening
with Max, talking, dancing or noticing changes in the tide. It
was one of those times which shine in the memory, but I
could not trust myself to relax even then. I had to take
control, go for the certainty of West Pluting, not . . .
Suddenly, I felt I should leave.

As though he sensed this, Max put his hand on mine. 'Can I see you again?'

'I'd like that, Max, but . . . '

'What's the matter?'

'It can't last, can it, in the circumstances.'

He leant back in his chair and gave a brief laugh. 'But we could still have some fun, couldn't we? We've got about . . . three weeks!'

I hesitated. 'Everything good ends. People move away. They die. Nothing lasts.'

'Oh, Vee, what a pessimistic outlook! Are you saying, then, that it's pointless doing anything because life is finite? What about carpe diem?'

'If I'm a pessimist, then I'm never disappointed. That's life. Anyway, I don't deserve you, Dr Greenwood.'

'Why? Because I'm so good-looking, accomplished – and modest . . .? Live a little, Vee. Let go, trust your instincts! Yes, we don't have long, but who knows where it might lead? We should make the best of the time we have left.'

We saw each other nearly every day for the next two weeks, and my soul sang with happiness and with the rightness of being with him. But as our parting grew nearer, I did not know how to convey my anxiety to Max, even when I had the chance. The fact remained that I was meant to be alone. I was a weak person who didn't deserve what Max seemed to be offering. His life was far too important to waste it with me. If I let things go on and he found out what I was really like, that would be it. The day before he was due to leave, we ended up at his flat with a Chinese takeaway. There were cases and boxes everywhere. I needed to try to explain.

'Max, I . . . don't think this is going to work.'

'What do you mean?'

'I can't miss this opportunity,' I replied quietly. 'It's not your fault. It's me. I can't do this. Sit down a minute and let's eat our food before it gets cold. I want to tell you something.'

We sat on the sofa and Max began unwrapping our meal on the table, putting out forks and a cloth for our fingers.

'Sorry, the other bits are packed.'

'It's alright.' I looked at him. 'I owe you an explanation. It involves a little story. Is that OK?'

'Go on then.'

'I remember when I was little, before Dad died, going to a fair with Mum. I don't know why, but we got there a bit late. It was just the two of us. I stood looking at all the brightly coloured stalls and watched a merry-go-round coming to a halt, with lots of flashing lights. The man in the blue cap and apron helped the last children down and they ran to their parents as he switched off all the lights. At that age, you're just a pair of eyes, aren't you?'

'Where's this leading, Vee?'

'Just then, I turned round to find Mum wasn't there. Where was she? I was terrified. I was alone in the darkening street, with litter blowing about. Then Mum appeared, and I burst into tears. "Oh, Vee!" she said, "I only went to get you a lolly before they closed!" Ever since then, if I see papers blowing around, I get a strangled feeling, as if I shouldn't be there on my own. I call it my "empty town" feeling. I don't need to see litter about, of course; I get the feeling as well when a market is packing up at the end of the day. Some of the stallholders are pulling down their clanging poles while others are shouting their last-minute bargains to a dwindling public. I always feel a sense of urgency, as if I should be getting home too, as if a storm is brewing.'

'I don't see what you're getting at.'

'I'm sure you can work out what the "empty town" feeling is; you're a doctor!'

'Maybe, but it's what it means *to you* that counts.'

I ate some of the food, then went on: 'I suppose it has to do with fear and wanting to be safe. I'm not saying I don't feel safe with you. Please don't think that. It's just that I feel I have to go with what . . . oh, I don't know how to explain it. All I know is it's got something to do with protecting myself in a world where, as I said before, Max, everything changes, everything ends.'

It would have been too strange to talk to him, of all

people, about black waves and white doors. After all, he wasn't my doctor and I wasn't about to submit to analysis. Sitting next to him on that old sofa felt right. I could not deny that, but then came the fear. We finished our meal in silence.

I felt a sudden impulse, even after trying to explain: 'I wish I could . . . I wish we were going away together,' I said cautiously.

'Oh, come with me then, Vee,' he said softly, as we kissed. 'Come with me to Edinburgh. I think I'm in –.'

' – Ssshh . . . don't . . . don't say it Max, please. I know.'

So he'd entered her life. He had no complaints about the way she'd told the story so far, but he hadn't yet found out what really happened in her next job, because they didn't see each other again after that evening; they simply went their separate ways. He had hoped she might come to the station to see him off. They spoke on the phone a couple of times, but they were not relaxed and things soon drifted.

Now he would hand this chapter to Helen, wondering how she would react to seeing him with Vee, who was about to start her new job. On with the story.

«*Les plaies du coeur guérissent mal.*
Souventes fois même, salut!
Elles ne se referment plus.»
GEORGES BRASSENS

10

Arnold College

'Are we still on for tonight?' I asked.

Patrick and I walked down the stairs together from the staffroom. Boys were not allowed upstairs, so they gathered in the foyer below to ask their questions or make their excuses when staff appeared.

'Yes, Vee. Come round about six.' Father Patrick Collins, the school chaplain, had taken me under his wing, it seemed.

'Sir, sir!'

'Bit late for homework now, isn't it, Perkins?' Patrick held the door open for me as I had a pile of books. Most of the men at Arnold College were considerate, but a few thought I was invading a male bastion. Though with Sixth Form girls now, they had to start appointing female staff; once again I was a pioneer, as I had been by going to university.

The classes here were larger and the marking took longer; that old feeling of inadequacy was stalking me, bringing back uncomfortable memories of my first school. But Thursday evenings at Patrick's lightened the atmosphere and also stopped me thinking too much about Max.

Patrick had a First from Cambridge and was also an expert cook. He had styled himself Father: he was not a Catholic. His flat was attached to one of the boarding houses, so I think my visits sparked some gossip among the boys. I walked into his white kitchen that evening.

'Hey! You'll never guess what Johnson came out with today!'

'Well, obviously not, so you're going to have to tell me.' He had a great line in playful sarcasm. His warm baritone and the stress he put on certain syllables, to the point of drawling, made his comments ring with irony and affection. The wine helped, too. I began chopping up some mushrooms for the sauce he was stirring. 'Well, go on then, tell me!'

I laughed. 'We were translating something into French and we needed to say, "I am back."'

Patrick put down his spoon, beckoned for me to add the mushrooms, then faced me, his hands braced on the worktop in mock suspense. 'Oh, God! I think I know what's coming!' He grimaced, removing his glasses and keeping just one eye open. 'Please put me out of my misery!'

I could hardly speak for laughing. 'He said, "je suis dos"!'

Patrick howled. 'I knew it! I knew it!'

This was our shared passion: words. Puns, jokes, dreadful translationese like this were everyday fare. Sometimes I think he made them up just for my benefit. He taught some Spanish but spoke fluent French as well, and his mediterranean appearance allowed him to pass as a native when he visited Spain every summer. I recognised the special look in his eyes for me, but it was all too often concealed by an actor's façade. There was a light which would vanish when noticed, leaving a touch of sadness as he looked away. He was proud to show me off when we ate at our favourite Indian restaurant, and he would take delight in teasing me in public, laughing at my red cheeks. At other times he could be very serious, even frosty, and our moods didn't always match up. And he never forgot he was a celibate priest.

Max was still on my mind although I hadn't spoken to him for a couple of weeks, but the fresh air Patrick brought into my life made Diane's party and the weeks with Max seem less real.

I didn't know it when I started work at Arnold College, but Max was still with me.

My periods had always been regular. But then I realised I was late, and my breasts felt heavy. So I bought a pregnancy test – and there it was: the result I had been dreading. I stared at it, trembling. Who could I talk to? I would tell Mum eventually, of course, but not until I had decided what to do. Patrick was not best placed to give advice. There were the house-mothers. No. It would be better if it was somebody outside school. I made an appointment to see a nurse at my GP's surgery.

'I've just found out I'm pregnant and I don't know what to do!' I blurted out.

Kathy raised her eyebrows, but otherwise her expression was controlled.

'Does the father know?'

'No. We . . . he's up in Edinburgh. We've both just started new jobs, and we're not seeing each other any more.'

'I see. Maybe if you t–.'

'–I don't want to upset his new life. He has a very important job.'

'So what help do you need from me?'

'I need to find out about having a termination.'

'Are you sure? I think you may need more time.'

'I've made up my mind. It's not the right time for me, even though I'm over thirty, and it's not the right time for . . . the father. He wouldn't be around and I couldn't do it, I mean, be a single mother. It would mess everything up.'

'What makes you say that?'

What I didn't tell the nurse was that I didn't *deserve* a baby at all. That night I told Mum and Ron, and the decision I'd reached. Ron said he would pay for it and we all met up at the clinic, which was halfway between West Pluting and Howcester. Mum was very quiet. The clinic was a bleak place, with strict procedures. I tried to detach myself from what was happening. It was half-term, so nobody at school needed to know.

Mum and Ron had seen me through university and never let me go without in terms of practical and emotional support. They had offered to drive me back home, which made it a very long round trip for them. Mum sat in the back, still quiet, but she massaged my shoulders.

'How do you feel, Vee?' Ron said, as we pulled out of the car park.

'Tired, but OK. Thanks for doing all this for me.'

'I'm here to help in any way I can.' We were stuck in traffic.

'I can't help wondering, though, if this wasn't my only chance to have a baby.'

'Oh, you'll get another chance, I'm sure. Don't worry, Vee.'

Hot tears ran down my face, suddenly and unexpectedly, as I thought of Max. I sobbed.

'Hey, hey, Vee! I'll pull over as soon as I can.' A couple of minutes later Ron stopped the car and put his arm round me. I let go of all my grief.

Back in West Pluting, alone in the cold flat, I wondered if I should ring Max. I decided not to. I'd arrived at the station on the day he left to see the train to Edinburgh pulling out. Then the phone rang.

'Vee? Are you alright? I've been trying to get you!'

'Oh, hello, Diane. I'm OK thanks. Sorry I haven't called you.'

'Yes, I should think so too! I've missed our weekly chats.'

'How're things with you and Jeff?'

'Oh, great thanks. We've had the house redecorated and . . . '

'And what?'

'Look, the Christmas holidays are nearly here. Why don't you come and stay for a couple of days when you break up? Not for Christmas itself, you understand – we'll have a houseful. But it'd be lovely to see you again and there's news to catch up on.'

I wanted to see Diane of course, but feeling as I did, I had to force myself to sound interested. I drove back along the coast to Lexby the day after the end of term. The boys' excitement in the lead up to Christmas, the concerts, shows, carols and Patrick's company hadn't moved me from my sense of loss. I hadn't told him, but he knew something was wrong. And I hadn't rung Max for weeks: I wasn't strong enough.

It was dark when I arrived at Diane's. It really was a magnificent house. The great sweeping staircase, with its red carpet and white banister, could be seen as soon as the door opened. She took my coat and showed me into the living room, where Jeff was putting the finishing touches to a large Christmas tree.

'I'll take you up to your room in a minute, but what can I get you? Cup of tea? Glass of mulled wine?' She rubbed her hands.

'Oh, that sounds good.'

Jeff climbed down the ladder. 'What d'you think? Will it do?'

I said it looked lovely, even though my heart just wasn't in it. 'How's business?'

'Not as good as it could be in the present climate, but we manage, don't we darling?'

Diane smiled as she brought in a tray with two glasses of wine and a cup of tea. She handed a glass to Jeff.

'Not having any wine, Diane?'

'No; I might later.'

'There's loads I want to ask you,' I said. 'How's the situation at the new place, Stonecastle?' We sat down.

Diane told how a couple of Castlebrough staff went there, including Joan Gibson, while the others either retired or moved on somewhere else. She suggested we drive round tomorrow and look at the site. The old school houses had to be demolished, which was a shame. But hey, she said, we would be in serious need of an appointment at the shops when we'd seen that! She smiled again. 'Got all your presents?'

'More or less. Are *you* at Stonecastle now?'

'No. That's one bit of news I've got for you. I was there, but I've just been made head of department over in East Brickham – last week in fact! For next term. Quite a drive, but I'm sure I'll love it! How's your new job going, Vee?'

'Oh, alright.' I felt a desperate need to unburden myself to her. 'But I've had a hard time lately because . . . '

Just then her phone rang, and as Diane bent over to pick

it up, I noticed something which made me very glad indeed that it had rung at that precise moment. It was only a short call, but it gave me the time to divert from my story, and spared my embarrassment.

'My sister. Anyway, what were you going to say, Vee?'

'Oh . . . it's just harder work where I am now. That's all.'

Diane patted the seat of the sofa next to her, indicating to Jeff that he should join her.

'We've got some other news, haven't we darling? Jeff smiled and placed his hand gently on Diane's stomach. 'Yes, you've guessed it. We're going to have a baby!'

'That's wonderful.' I was pleased for them, but I ached inside. 'When's it due?'

'In May. We were planning to get married first, but then we had this little surprise. So the wedding's on hold for now, but it will happen, and you'll be invited.' Her face was lit with happiness. 'By the way, Vee – have you kept in touch with Max at all?'

January brought gales and sleet. I looked out of the staffroom window at the moorland sky. Clouds trailed their unstitched hems over the city, the grey sustained by the granite and concrete of its post-war reconstruction. In the distance, beyond the rugby pitch, condensed rows of houses were interspersed with the black trunks and branches of leafless trees.

Mr Green came in at the start of my free lesson and set all the notices on the board fluttering in the draught. 'Rachel Mills is downstairs for you, Vee.'

I put my coffee on the table and moaned. 'She's probably forgotten her book or something.' Hail was rattling on the roof and bouncing on the grass. Rachel did not look at me properly when I went down the stairs. Instead she turned away, her head down, her long dark hair falling loose in its band and her arms folded. 'Rachel?'

'Miss.' She was trying not to cry.

'What's wrong?'

'Can I . . . can I talk to you? I mean, is it OK now?'

'Let's find a free room.' We waited for the weather to ease a bit, then dashed across to the next building. Room 7 was empty. There was a long silence while Rachel composed herself. I gave her a tissue, then attempted to reduce the noise of the weather by closing the sash window. We sat on grey plastic chairs and our voices echoed slightly because of the high ceiling.

'Miss, it's my mum. She's ill. They took her away last night. She had to be . . . sectioned, I think that's what they called it. She's been acting really strange for a while, but Dad and I didn't know what was wrong. We were so frightened. My little sister locked herself in her room . . . '

'Oh, Rachel. I'm so sorry. Is there anything I can do?'

'I don't think so Miss. I just needed to talk to someone, you know. You won't tell anyone else, will you? Only if it gets out my Mum is a nutcase, my life won't be worth living.'

'I won't say anything if you don't want me to – and I certainly wouldn't use that kind of word. If there's a problem, I'll say you're not feeling well or something. But just remember, Rachel: she's still your mum and she will get better.'

I had to move to a different flat for the third time in two years. Patrick helped me on this occasion (not that I had much to move) because the new place, number 79, was only ten minutes' walk from Arnold College.

We were seeing each other more often outside school. I pressed the button on his entryphone and announced, 'C'est moi!' as usual. The door buzzed and I went in. Sitting on the steps in front of Patrick's door was Leo McPherson, head in hands.

'Did you want Father Collins?' I asked.

The young boy nodded. When Patrick came to his door, combing his hair in apparent anticipation of our Indian meal in town, I drew my hand silently across my throat and grimaced, pointing to McPherson.

'Hello, Mac. Do you want to come in?' McPherson stood up without a word. He looked pale and tired.

'Come in and tell me what's happened.' Patrick's voice was warm and he showed the boy into the small living room with its old-fashioned furniture. I sat next to Leo on the sofa.

'Sir . . . Miss,' came a tiny voice. 'It's my dad. He had an accident and . . . ' At this point Leo burst into tears and screamed: 'He's dead!'

I put my arm round the boy. Then Patrick indicated, with his eyebrows and a jerk of his head, that he wanted a word outside. 'I'm really sorry about this, Gatters,' he murmured. 'But just before all this I had a phone call from a friend who's in trouble and I said I'd call in. So we'll have to forego supper this time and . . . will you be alright to stay with Mac for about an hour?'

'Yes, OK.'

He smiled and squeezed my hand. 'If you get hungry there's stuff in the fridge.'

I made us a sandwich at some point and I sat with Leo until ten o'clock, when his housemaster rang, anxious. I put him in the picture and sent the boy downstairs. His mother was going to collect him in the morning. Shortly afterwards, Patrick returned. He poured us a glass of wine each and flopped into the sofa next to me with a sigh of exhaustion. A few moments passed. He ran his fingers through his hair.

'Makes you think, Vee, doesn't it, about taking your parents for granted. What I need is a wife. You could be Mrs Collins, then . . . '

I cut him short with a passionate kiss that had been waiting for months. But he sat up and gently pulled away from me. I ran out of the flat. Patrick and I did not speak for several months. When we eventually rescued our friendship, it was subtly changed, like a fine plate with a chip which we couldn't help noticing.

11

Falling

Spring: the earth was waking up, delicately green. But I was spending more and more time in my own private weird season. Spring was too industrious for me and sent a kind of muted panic through my bones. I could hear the exam bird, the chaffinch, growing ever more insistent. I was angry with myself because I kept getting things wrong; this feeling would then fade into a grey apathy, because nothing could be done about it.

I know I must have interrupted other teachers talking about me when I went into the staffroom. The slight turn of their backs and the repeated parcels of silence gave it away. Some of my classes were misbehaving and I couldn't keep up with the marking. I never knew which teacher had been in the next room at any given time; this undermined my confidence. The senior staff were beginning to ask questions. The black wave was threatening. I remembered my first job, but no amount of determination could change the way I felt.

I spent days in bed. I didn't clean the flat at the weekend as I normally did. It was the monochrome, the black threat, the weakness of university. I think Aunt Mary was awake. When I did manage to go into work, sometimes it felt as if I was just a mask walking along and trying to teach. If the mask were to fall off, there would be nobody behind it. And it was a poor, brittle mask. Then suddenly my lessons would go brilliantly, the world would be wonderful, full of light and energy. I'd hardly need any sleep and my thoughts and ideas would come so, so easily. It was a shame my classes did not share my enthusiasm: I was angry at this. Then came a phase when all I wanted to do was drive off a cliff or take an overdose. Either this notion would fill my head, or my mind would be empty and dark. Whichever it was, I would sit in front of my students and not engage with them. How they could be expected to tolerate this erratic behaviour I don't know; right then, however, their welfare couldn't have been further from my mind. And now it had all ground to a halt. The urge to end the moods once and for all was still there but I hadn't the strength to see it through.

I didn't know how long I'd been alone in the flat. One moment I'd been trying to get people at school to sponsor me for a Channel swim, the next I couldn't even get in the bath.

A sharp knock at the door broke into my curtained world.

'Oh . . . Gatters!' Patrick was looking at a face I hadn't seen for a while and he had to smile quickly to hide his reaction. 'Can I come in?'

He followed me along the passage to the kitchen. Until then, I had not let anyone see me without make-up, but now I didn't care. Everything had sunk inside me to its lowest level. I had no resistance, no opinion, no emotion. Patrick coughed and we sat on the pine chairs. His jacket sparkled with drops of rain and he brought a school smell with him which sent a wave of guilt and anxiety through me. He took off his glasses and wiped them clean. There was concern in his voice.

'Have you been to see Keith?' We had the same GP.

I shook my head. Speaking was an effort.

'Only . . . ' He coughed again. 'I think you should, my dear. Because I think you're depressed.' There was that word. I hadn't heard it for a while.'Do you want me to come with you?'

'Across the Channel?'

'No, Vee. To see the doctor.'

'I don't know.'

Patrick sighed. 'They're worried about you at the College. Please let me drive you down to see Keith.'

His will was there, still strong; mine had evaporated.

There was only his to follow.

'It would be a good idea if you had a bath before we go, I think,' he said kindly. 'I'll wait in the living room, shall I, while you do that, yes?'

A moment later, as I went towards the bathroom, I heard curtains being jerked open.

We sat in the dimly-lit cell that was the doctors' waiting room.

'Vee Gates?' came a voice. It was becoming more and more difficult to move, but I stood up and managed to get into Dr Mann's room with Patrick's help.

'Hello, Vee.' Dr Mann shone his grey eyes at me over his glasses. His gaze was almost painful and I looked at my knees. He must be able to see into me, see what a weak person I am. 'Do you mind Patrick being here?' I shake my head. I sense that Dr Mann and Patrick are looking at each other, because I recognise a parcel of silence despite the blackness.

'How do you feel?'

It is like being asked to speak a foreign language. 'Can't . . . describe. Grey.'

'Do you think you are depressed?'

That word again. I nod. 'Worse . . . than at uni . . . '

'Would you like to see a psychiatrist?'

Something melts in me and I want to cry, but I can't. The only psychiatrist I want to see right now is Max. But the word "psychiatrist" tells me it is the beginning of the end. I am worthless. I'm not even worth all this effort from them. Patrick moves his hand as if he is about to put it on my arm, then thinks better of it. He mutters something about letting Mum know, then he and Dr Mann have a short conversation.

Not caring what they say is a bit like being a child again.

'I think you should go into hospital, Vee,' Dr Mann says in the end. 'I'll make the arrangements. You go home and put a few things in a bag. Patrick's offered to drive you over there.'

'Not . . . like a dog . . . on a lead!' It is the old nightmare
and I am Aunt Mary. I am afraid and intensely fragile. I don't
know what to expect or how I am going to deal with this. I
haven't mentioned Aunt Mary to Patrick. Why are they
being so nice to me? I am angry because I am failing, so why
aren't *they* angry with me? Then I see it. The white door is
swinging open, the padlock hanging by a curved metal
finger, and a black tunnel appears; I can hear the echo of
rows of black doors closing sharply along it, like an old train
about to leave. An angry voice repeats that I am useless. The
white door, the whole building, seems to be moving slightly,
up and down, and getting larger, filling the world. The ivy
is now blue, sparking, electrified.

Then I realise that I am the one who is moving towards it,
towards its black tunnel, but I am beyond fear. I am powerless, as in a dream, pulled in and pushed along by the black
wave. A face appears, speaking, but I cannot understand the
words. The tunnel opens out inside and there are people
walking and sitting. The carpet is stained and I can smell
tobacco and disinfectant. Someone is asking me questions in
a quiet place with soft chairs. I try to answer, but my voice
is slow and old. Then I hear a different voice which leads me
along a corridor with a lot of noise. Walking is difficult. I
follow a pair of shoes which has to slow down. An arm
points to a bed in a small room.

The first night, everything moved into a different
perspective, a kind of flat inevitability. Resignation,
surrender, but without effort. All the possibilities of my life
were reduced to a black dot, a single point in time, where I
was completely and inescapably alone.

I am a grey slab floating on a dark sea. I can see nothing,
feel nothing except a warm rush sometimes between my
legs. I am not asleep, nor am I awake. The black wave takes
me along and I cannot move, cannot choose where I am
going. My head is a black screen and I cannot tell if I have a
body. There seems to be some kind of awareness behind the
screen, but I don't know if the awareness is part of me.
Sometimes I think I hear a voice in the distance and some-

times it seems possible that people are touching me, but then I am alone again on the dark sea for an eternity.

A crack appears to the right of my black screen. One eye has opened and light is coming in. Like tuning an old TV set, both eyes then try to adjust to a different channel, a different reality. The picture is blurred and I remember my glasses, but I have no idea where they are.

This is not my bedroom. My head aches. I don't know where I am or how long I've been here. Somebody is sitting in a chair outside the door; she gets up when she hears me try to speak. I cough, then feel weak and lie staring at the irregular pattern of the ceiling tiles. The person has disappeared. I sleep for a while. When I wake up, everything is still grey and grainy, but I think I hear Max's voice. Or is it Jim's? Someone is sitting in the chair by my bed. I still find it hard to understand what he or she is saying, but I pick out the word "water" and nod my head. The liquid is passing through my mouth and throat as if it were my first ever drink.

At least I know I have a body now, if only because it has no strength. The person is talking to me, explaining something. They want me to sign a piece of paper. I notice bags of clothes on the floor, a vase of flowers. They don't look real.

I sleep, wake and sleep again. It might be another day. Now I am being taken somewhere in a wheelchair, up in a lift and along a corridor with a different coloured carpet, my head bent forward. Blue things. The voice is telling me I'm useless and I cannot question what is happening. We arrive at another small room. I am told to lie on a black bed. There are three or four people in the room and some equipment.

Someone opens my dressing gown and puts stickers and wires on my chest. A needle is inserted into the back of my hand, then I hear the hiss of the oxygen mask.

They put it over my face . . .

Oh, God, Vee, he thought. He wished he'd been there. He felt terrible. He had a pain.

'Darling, are you alright? You're very quiet this evening.' Helen took the plates away. 'I think you're spending too long on the book. What've you read?'

He couldn't answer properly. He had not seen the meal in front of him that night. All he could see was Vee's book on his desk, open at the next chapter Helen would read. She thought he'd been overdoing it, but he was in a state of shock.

A baby! And then that description . . . Back in the attic, he felt a sudden anger. He wanted to trash the room, and the only thing that stopped him was the thought of Helen's reaction. Why hadn't Vee told him about being pregnant? They needn't have parted; she had really wanted to go with him to Edinburgh, hadn't she? He found himself panting, walking to and fro, wringing his hands, trying not to scream out, squeezing his head. They could have brought up the child together. And even if she didn't want it, she could at least have *told* him! He brought his fist down hard on the desk. Then his eyes filled with tears and he found he was sobbing. But he couldn't share this with Helen, not right now, and certainly not with Simon, who seemed to be drinking too much. So he tried to pull himself together. How different his life would have been! Though he couldn't imagine not having Grace and Anna – or Helen. He wasn't aware just how much he *needed* to be involved in helping Vee until then. Oh! A gripping pain and he dropped to his knees . . .

'I came up to ask you if . . . Max! Are you alright? Oh my God. Simon! Simon! Max is having a heart attack. Get an ambulance!'

12

Moods

Despite her anxiety, Helen wanted to read what Max had read before his collapse. She took the relevant chapters to the hospital; it was something to do while she was waiting, sitting by his bed. Then she continued reading beyond that.

They took me to the black bed and the mask several times. Time lost its meaning: it was something other people controlled. I was bathed. I was fed some jelly, with a spoon, like a baby. They gave me tablets every day.

Once, as I walked along in my nightdress, they were watching me in the irregular corners of my vision and I didn't know why. I heard a voice making a strange noise, then realised it was mine. Not the same voice which came to me in the dark times, telling me I was useless, scorning my every move, showing me I could do nothing right, filling my head with expletives and deserved derision as if I had head-phones – no, these sounds were different and came from my mouth. Then the nurses began talking about me as if I couldn't hear. I was being steered, even though nobody touched me, back into my room. A scream erupted from me and I was suddenly strong and unbearably angry. I set about destroying the room and then I was grabbed and put on the bed. A sharp sting in my bottom, then I was crying, panting, held still for a moment. The anger faded. I lay half asleep. But my soul-pain was still there. I knew it would not stop until after I had more ECT or until I died.

These were the two Black Posts I clung to: ECT and Death. The intensity of each moment had to be escaped and the two

Black Posts were all I had. Nothing else mattered. I dreaded losing hold of them. I had to have one in each hand all the time and I couldn't let anyone take them away. Anything anyone did was likely to disturb them and I couldn't bear the idea of a single word doing that much damage. I was lying on a flat stone in a black desert, pinned there by the wave, now lapping quiet and congealed, as I waited to find out which of my posts would be stronger.

Suddenly I had a new, bright red tide in my head, mixed with the black. The two strands, black then red – well, really they were ropes to pull on, but I could never find the ends – took me one way, then another, like driftwood.

Strange world. No sandwich. Blue things. Yes I know I'm useless. You keep telling me. I know. Nurses watching me. Doctor talking to me. Sitting. Can't speak. Elbows on knees, hiding face. Slow. Colours strange. Blue things. Trying to walk. Can't feel anything. Brain is black hole. Yes I know. Hate myself. Want to die. Would do it if had energy. Must deserve it. I'm useless, I know. They're watching, on edge of my screen. No food. Hide my head. I'm useless . . . NOW! ENERGY! Oh, hello, nurse – you're Steve, aren't you? Pleased to meet you! – Now I must dance, and all these other people must dance too! I'll teach them what REAL dancing's all about! Why do they look at me like that? – Why so down, Cam? – Don't give a damn, Cam! – Don't be like a lamb, Sam! – Hahahaha! – I have lots of plans for this hospital, but I haven't got time to discuss that with you right now – can't stop – think I'll get a Mercedes like that – I'll go into town tomorrow – I like dancing – wheee! J'aime danser – et chanter – don't want to stop or go to my room. Bet I could teach you a thing or two in my room, eh Steve? Nudge, nudge, say na more!.. FALLING. Must sit down. Speed of falling – brain shrivelling. Can't be seen. Hide my face. Not a real person. Not worth anything. Can't control it. Yes I know I'm useless. Feel guilty. Am nothing. Deserve to die . . .

Then one day it was time to speak to the psychiatrist.

'Vee? Doctor Wilson will see you now.'

As I walk slowly into the room, I am aware that several other people besides the doctor are there, sitting in a semi-circle, with him in the middle, at the top, under the window.

'Well, Vee. How do you feel now after some ECT?' The doctor's bald head is shining.

'I . . . think I feel a bit better. But what has been going on? Is that what a breakdown's like?'

'You have been having mood swings. It's not simple depression as we first thought, but manic depression. Rapid cycling.' At least there was a name for it, I thought, looking at my knees. And at least I could now string a sentence together.

'You have two more treatments next week, which should improve things even more. We've put you on lithium. There are leaflets about that; just ask the nurses. Any questions?'

'No.' Doctors don't have that much time. When I left the ward round, Kit, a foreign nurse, came up to me and said I had a visitor. Disguising his reaction to me just as Patrick had done when he came to my flat at the start of it all, the headmaster of Arnold College was waiting in the visitors' room.

'Hello, Vee. How are you?' his voice boomed.

'Not too bad.'

'Look, Vee, I won't beat about the bush. I think it's time we called it a day, don't you?'

Patrick had crept into the room in front of him a moment earlier. He had brought me some flowers but did not take part in this: he couldn't change what had been decided. The headmaster left.

'Why haven't you been before, Patrick?' I sobbed.

'I *have* been before – twice, in fact!' Patrick sounded almost insulted, but immediately calmed his voice. 'Well actually, I'm not really surprised you don't remember. You were very ill.'

'The ECT has affected my memory, too.' I tried to stop crying. 'I don't know if you ever get this, but I have a kind of *feeling* that a memory exists, without being able to say what it is. It's as if some memories are trying to reach me from behind a curtain. It's a bit like when you're hunting for a particular word.'

'I know that one!'

'Oh, but I'm so tired. I'm sorry, Patrick, but I'm going to have to sleep now.'

When he had gone, I realised that I'd actually been crying: I hadn't been able to until then. A strange progress to wish for. And the hostile voice in my head was gone for the moment, at least. It was as if the black wave, which I could hardly remember now, had been washed away with clear water. I slept. I always had to sleep for some time after ECT as well, and usually woke up with a headache and too late for lunch.

Patrick came back the following week.

'Why do I have this feeling I've lost my job?' I was puzzled by the nagging thought.

Patrick coughed and was obviously trying to think how to answer.

'I have, haven't I? You know something I don't! What's happening, Patrick?'

'Don't you remember the headmaster's visit last week?'

'No.'

'Well, he . . . er . . . He said, "I think it's time we called it a day".'

'So it's true then.' I felt empty.

I was shocked to see a grey, pinched face looking at me from the mirror. The real me. I washed, then decided it was time to ask the nurses some questions. 'Ian, have you got a moment?'

'What's up, Vee?'

'I need you to help me sort some things out in my head.'

'Right. I'll be with you in one minute. Wait here.'

I stood outside the nurses' office on the dirty carpet.

'Now, shall we talk in your room?' I had formed a bond with Ian, the most approachable of the nurses and I felt stressed when he wasn't on duty.

'Ian – how long have I been here?'

'You've been on Tor ward, oooh, about six weeks.'

'As long as that!' Suddenly I realised that I had not lived part of my own life.

'You were very unwell when you arrived and you went – d'you want me to explain what happened?'

'Please.'

'You went into what's called stupor for over a week. We were worried about you because you didn't eat at all then. When you came out of that, your moods started swinging violently; you had eight or nine "ups" and eight or nine "downs" in a day! Then you started a course of ECT, twice a week, and I think I'm right in saying that you've only got one treatment left.'

'That's right. How many's that?'

'That will be ten.'

'Do you think I'm better now? I can't really tell.'

'Oh, I should say so! The ECT has made a massive difference. You could hardly speak or walk.'

'But now I've lost my job.'

'That's bad luck. But Vee, people don't understand mental illness. They read a newspaper report about someone having been murdered by an "axe-wielding psychopath" and they think that everybody with mental health issues is like that. They don't consider the possibility,' he went on, with an exasperated smile, 'that the sufferer is actually *more* afraid than they are. And they conveniently overlook their own aunt, or whoever, who's not well, because that can't *possibly* be part of the same thing, can it? The main thing, though, is that they can't see that people don't *choose* to be ill. I mean, did *you* choose what's happened to you? But, hey, listen to me going on!'

'Will it . . . will it happen again?'

'Impossible to predict. Some people only ever have one episode. Others get ill again if they stop taking their meds. Others again take their meds but *still* have a series of episodes.'

'So you can't say which I'll be. But Ian, why has this happened to me? I must be weak and useless.'

'It can be hereditary.' He slapped both hands on his thighs. 'Vee, I must go. I'm sorry I can't be more helpful. Medication everybody!'

In the queue forming along the corridor, I joined the ranks of those I once despised.

The sun shone between the tall trees lining the main drive up to the old hospital buildings. It was my first time outside and I had found that my clothes were quite loose. Ian came with us. I was a bit high at the time and I laughed at Barbara, who was walking really slowly.

Inside the door with flaking navy paint was a dingy café. We sat in a corner with our green NHS cups and saucers. Ian said he'd be back in ten minutes.

Some strange characters inhabited this world. A shaft of light from a high window cut a sample of the smoky air, and we watched in silence as a man of about forty-five walked to and fro, in and out of this spotlight, keeping up a loud replay of the latest conversation with his psychiatrist, speaking both parts. Every so often he would go up to the counter and buy a single cigarette. His eyes saw only the bits of the real world he needed at any given moment. The rest of the time, he was totally immersed in his private dialogue made public. Another man sat nearby, in drab clothes, chain-smoking as if with a mechanical arm, rocking back and forth on his chair, his lips moving silently the whole time, saliva trickling down his chin, adding to the dark patch on the lapel of his jacket.

They were long-stay patients from Albert ward, up here in the original asylum, but they seemed to be from a different century. A bent old woman shuffled round on a tour of the ashtrays, looking for decent butts. To make a new cigarette, she would crumble the tobacco from the butts onto a paper and roll it up. I had seen people doing this on Tor ward as well. Not only did these people from Albert have very little money – fags were the patients' currency – they never seemed to have visitors to bring them anything. Did they *have* anyone? Did anybody know they were there? Had they been abandoned, years ago? They made me think of old slanting gravestones, neglected and forgotten.

By the time we had finished our tea my mood had changed again. Ian and Barbara had to support me down the hill and back to Tor ward. The swings were not as frequent or as intense though by now, and at least I was more aware of those around me.

I was getting wise to things that happened on Tor ward as well. The whole of society was represented, but as if in parody. I became able to work out why the other patients were there. The ones who did not appear to be ill were ready for discharge. You had to know whom you could trust to go to the shop for you, too. I wanted a cigarette.

'Oh, here she comes! Just 'cos she's having ECT, she thinks she's special. And did you hear her the other day, when she was high, bragging about her degree!'

'I know, she's the big "I am". Makes me sick. So up herself.'

I realised I must have embarrassed myself when I was in the grip of this thing, but no more so than others I'd met on the ward, who gave completely the wrong impression of what they were like in the real world. Seeing them get better proved this. They became calmer, quieter and most of all, their features seemed to shrink back to a normal size from the cartoon version they had come in with. I couldn't help thinking of Aunt Mary's rolling eyes.

I decided not to sit in the smoking room after all; I went into the garden. Gil was sitting on one of the benches. He was a quiet friend, a companion in depression. As I walked towards him, he raised his eyes. They were concentration-camp eyes, hollow but shining with an invincible light.

The last one: nothing to eat or drink after midnight, blood pressure check in the morning, hand in your valuables and write "bag in office" on your hand to avoid alarm when you come round. It's hard to believe, but it's things like that you forget. Wait til you're sent for, then up the back stairs with your assigned nurse to the ECT suite.

There is the black bed again. The room is full of equipment and there is the doctor, a nurse and the anaesthetist.
Climb on the bed – a trolley, I now realise. Any caps or
crowns? No. Leads on my chest, pulse monitor on my finger,
find a vein. I feel cold today and it makes it harder for them
to find one. Scratch: now the valve is in my hand. A cold
trickle runs up inside to my elbow. Oxygen mask and . . .

I've missed you Mum.' We hugged each other. Then we sat
in the living room at number 79, two days after I had been
discharged from Tor ward. The grass was long and I only
had two tea bags left. 'How's Jim?'

'Oh fine. I think he's got a new girlfriend, but I'd better let
him tell you himself.'

We drank our tea. The old clock I had bought ticked on.

'Vee, I'm really sorry I couldn't visit you in hospital, but
it's a long way to come, and the main reason is of course that
Ron's been so ill. Flu then pneumonia. I couldn't leave him
and I couldn't tell you at the time. I was so relieved to hear
your voice on the phone the other day though, sounding
more like your old self. And Ron's made a full recovery. So
my dear people are back with me.'

I tried to explain how strange I felt: I didn't really know
who my old self was any more. Assuming of course that
people have constant "selves" to which they can return.
From what? Where had I been then, in the meantime, if I
wasn't with my self?

I told Mum that one of the nurses out there had said this
might be hereditary. This did not come as such a shock to
Mum, thank goodness, although neither of us could work
out why, if that were the case, *she* hadn't been affected. If
some crisis was needed to "switch on" the illness, surely
Dad's death would have done it? But she was more interested in learning all about ECT.

'Well, you're put to sleep – see the little scars on my hand?
Then they put a *small* electric current through your brain.'

'Oh, I don't like the sound of that!'

'But it is only a small amount. You have a kind of fit, but you don't know about it of course, then you wake up.'

Mum pulled a face. I explained that not everybody has this treatment, and anyway, it doesn't always work for those who *do* have it. In fact, I went on, nobody really knows how it works in the first place, but then again, they don't always know how the tablets work either. As she could see though, it had worked for me, and that's all that mattered for now. I said I didn't know if I'd be there today if wasn't for ECT. OK, it had affected my memory, but they'd told me a lot would come back.

She stood up. 'Right, are we going shopping or not? You need a lampshade for the hall for one thing. I was shocked when I got here last night to see a bare bulb!' She bought me a tee shirt and lunch as well, and we restocked the kitchen.

'I'll stay one more night, Vee.'

We set about cooking a meal, while I tried to tell her what things were like in Tor ward and how I felt, but it sounded false and unreal, as if I was recounting a nightmare which nobody else could understand because they hadn't lived through it. Or perhaps it was somebody else's nightmare. But every attempt to describe what I had in fact only *half* lived was inadequate. You don't experience psychosis; it's the nature of the beast. So I don't think Mum was any the wiser in the end. And I could appreciate why people find illness like this so hard to understand. If those who experience it can't describe it properly, what hope is there?

'So what are you going to do about work then, Vee?'

'Oh, don't remind me. The money I got from the College won't last forever, so I'll have to start looking soon I suppose. Something tells me it might take a while.'

13

Aftershocks

Lucy Bennett had a tiny office overlooking the car park. The clinic on the hill was surrounded by trees planted when it was built and it reminded me of my old school. Her room was full of books, leaving just enough space for a desk and two chairs.

'Now, you've been referred to me after your recent admission to Tor ward.' Her hazel eyes smiled at me. She had an oval face and shortish greying hair, from which long thin russet-coloured earrings emerged, toning with her unusual jacket. 'Do you know why you're here?'

'Not really.'

'Well, a psychologist's job is to try to unravel any thought patterns which might have contributed to your becoming ill. Of course you'll go on seeing Dr Wilson as well.'

'I see.'

'What I think would be helpful,' she went on, 'for both of us, is if you keep a diary of your moods, and bring it to our next session in a fortnight.'

I nodded. Using the glasses on a chain round her neck, Lucy glanced briefly at her notes, making her earrings move.

'So, Vee, how do you feel now?'

'There are gaps in my memory which can be awkward. Apart from that, I don't really know how I feel. It changes from day to day. I don't know if I'm the same person as I used to be before I was ill, or whether I'm on my way back and haven't got there yet. I suppose only time will tell.'

'Try and capture these states of mind in your mood diary. Do you keep a diary anyway?'

'Yes.'

'Good. What about your moods, specifically. Do you think they've settled down?'

'Well I don't feel as weird as I did. I feel more or less level, just a bit wrung out.'

'Do you feel able to talk about your father? When did he die?'

I hadn't seen Patrick for a while, but then it *was* exam time. For a week or two all I wanted to do was sleep, but I knew I had to make an effort to get a job. I arranged to meet up with one of the men I'd flirted with when high in hospital, but realised immediately that I shouldn't have done. In our normal lives, we wouldn't have given each other a second glance. I could tell he felt the same; I vowed I would never make the same mistake again.

Then one evening, there was a knock at the door. To my surprise, Ian the nurse was standing there, in cycling helmet and gloves, holding the handlebars of a racing bike, which he was trying to prop against the porch wall.

'I've done something I shouldn't have,' he said quietly. 'I looked up your address in the notes.'

'Come in,' I said, eyeing his lycra shorts and muscular legs and imagining . . . well. 'Cup of tea?' I asked, as if trying to deny what was in the air.

'Great. How are you?' We went into the living room.

'OK I think.'

He smiled. I stood for a moment, looking at him, and felt a silly, matching smile grow on my lips from the tension, which had to be broken. But by whom? Getting the tea was my way of opting out, although of course I would have to come back. But Ian followed me through into the kitchen. I put the mugs out and his hand was on my shoulder. I thought any feelings I might have had towards him had died when I left the ward, but I was wrong.

'This has to stay between you and me, yes?' he said softly into my neck. I turned and we kissed. The kettle boiled unnoticed as our desire exploded and we found ourselves undressing at top speed and landing on the bed. We went at it like animals.

Ian came round once a week for two or three months, but the lust soon faded. We couldn't go out anywhere as a couple; it was like being with Tony. So once we had discovered each other's bodies, there was nothing left to do. He could lose his job if he wasn't careful. So we went our separate ways.

At my appointment with Dr Wilson, he said I should stay on lithium, with regular blood tests which I had to arrange. Then a letter came about a course I was required to attend to get me back to work. Such things were in their infancy.

Charmian Davies ran the course, held weekly in a dingy office in town. There were about eight of us, mostly men, in the cramped room. It didn't take me long to realise that the course was designed for people with poor literacy skills, who didn't have the first idea about how to apply for jobs or speak on the phone. Although unimpressed by the first session, I decided to give it another week or two, in case I missed something useful. But the content of Charmian's next two stints left me cold. In fact, I was angry, because she used me. She had recognised that I didn't need to be there. So she used me.

'I'm not coming back!'

Charmian looked at me in alarm, her painted eyebrows resembling a clown's. I heard the door creak as the others left. 'But Vee . . . you've got to!'

'Look, I know how to write a letter and speak on the phone, as you well know. I came here to get help, but so far I've just been helping *you* to help those other people. And I'm not even getting paid for it! Besides which, it's insulting. Just because I'm unemployed doesn't mean I can't think!' With that, I stormed out and walked the mile back to number 79 in the rain and the wet leaves.

The next day I bought newspapers, writing paper, envelopes and stamps. This was in the days before the

Internet. Just me and the kitchen table; so, the great task began. It seemed I would have to do it on my own, as Charmian wasn't much use.

Every day without fail for the next two years I wrote and sent off at least two applications. There was no proper system for finding work in those days. You signed on and were left to your own devices.

I took the whole thing seriously, starting by looking only at jobs for graduates, but I quickly formed the impression that employers had closed ranks on me. At the same time, I realised that I didn't have to be quite so honest about my problems on paper. But even then, the watered-down "occasional depression" on medical questionnaires was enough for a rejection. Time was passing, the money was running out, I'd only had three interviews in eight months and I knew I'd have to start applying for jobs which did not require a degree. Getting a job had been a simple task before and I couldn't understand why it was suddenly so difficult. Then I realised that this was stigma in action, and it hurt.

Meanwhile I wanted to find out about manic depression as well. It seemed that most people diagnosed with it had a sustained episode of one mood or the other. There were dozens of different medications; new types appeared every so often. The discovery that I was in good company – a large number of artists, writers and other famous and creative people had this diagnosis – was cold comfort in my present circumstances.

The person I really needed to know about was Aunt Mary. Mum said she'd been in hospital in Oxford, but that's all she knew. Things like this just weren't discussed at the time, and the Wheeler family would have been in disgrace socially if anyone had found out. Mum had obviously done some research of her own. Did I realise, she asked, that unmarried mothers were incarcerated for years too? Prejudice against women was nowhere near as bad as it used to be, she thought. In her view, I should count myself lucky that we lived in more enlightened times; I had no evidence that we did.

I made some phone calls and discovered that Mary Wheeler had been admitted to George ward in 1912, aged twenty, with "acute delirious mania". She had three further episodes of illness. Then, in 1939, she committed suicide.

I looked into my mind: the white door had closed again, but the padlock had disappeared. Whether this was dangerous remained to be seen.

When Max came out of hospital – he didn't remember much about the heart attack except the pain – he was under strict instructions not to overdo things and take gentle exercise. Helen had of course been reading the book; she was surprisingly calm. She came and sat on the bed. He was allowed to get up late nowadays. At Helen's urgent request, Simon had given Jackson a good talking-to at last it seemed, about the noise at night. Helen really wanted the two of them out.

There were two get-well cards, from Grace and Anna. Helen had phoned them when he went in, and they had been ready to come home if necessary, as Helen put it.

'But hey! Max, you really loved Vee, didn't you?' She smiled. 'I know you told me about her, but it was still interesting to read Vee's version.'

He felt she deserved an explanation. 'Helen, I want you to understand that I swear I knew nothing about the pregnancy until I read that chapter myself.'

She stroked his head. 'I know, darling. I believe you. Your heart attack was proof enough of that. I'm just glad you're OK. And now I've gone on ahead of you with the reading, so you've some catching up to do!'

That was the only thing he really felt like doing. He didn't think there could be any more surprises concerning him in Vee's book. He asked Helen what she thought had driven Vee to suicide.

'Hold on. I need to get things clear in my mind. First, Max, I never did ask you properly what your motives are for doing this. I mean, you're retired, we could be on holiday, cough, cough, hint, hint. Vee's dead . . . Why do you, specifically, need to go into what happened at Squaremile? Because it looks as though that's where we're headed. Yes, I said I'd help, but – .'

'– I want to do something to help people like Vee in the future. And I abhor stigma and discrimination. That's my motivation. I'm still a doctor really. It's often quoted, and I'm sure you've heard it, but Burke was meant to have said something like, "It is necessary only for the good man to do nothing for evil to triumph". You might have got there, but I haven't reached the point in her book when she became my patient; I saw the damage the illness did to Vee and the changes it brought about in her life. It may never be possible to know the full extent of someone's suffering, but I believe Vee did ask for my help.'

'And you felt guilty. I know that. I remember working that out at the funeral.'

'I did feel guilty. So, what drove her to commit suicide?'

Helen thought for a moment. 'Vee lost things. Important things.' She paused to stroke his head again. 'People and things she'd loved or put effort into. In the end, she must have thought she'd lost everything. That's the answer to your question: loss. The rest of her book will bear this out, I'm sure.'

14

Squaremile

During the two years in West Pluting I spent looking for work, I got to know every knot, ring and repair in that kitchen table. It was the scene of triumph and despair (mostly the latter), of hours of careful writing rewarded by a standard letter of rejection – or, frustratingly, by no response at all, which at first I considered rude, but then became resigned to. I kept a careful written record.

As I said, this was before the Internet. The post usually brought disappointment. An invitation to interview was an excuse to open a bottle of wine, but stigma usually won the day, even if I did get an interview. I never went into detail about my illness, but if the subject came up, the look in people's eyes told me that it was all over; they hardly needed to say anything. A kind of shutter descended and I knew that was it. Sadly, the law which requires you to declare your disability is the very one which seals your fate. Discrimination has the last word when, having exhausted all possibilities for employment, you are likely to be looked down on, *blamed* for not working; people don't see the connection with their own attitude: "You ought to be working. You're just lazy. But *we* won't employ you. And nor will anyone else".

At the end of May, however, I had two phone calls, both with some good news. The first was from Lexby: a proud Jeff announced that mother and son, all 8lb 10oz of him, were doing fine, and so I decided to visit Diane again while I still had a car. But I felt as if we had all moved on, as if I had picked up a handful of sand and it had run through my fingers, with a sagging, mocking, trombone diminuendo in my head which told me I should really be aware that things had changed, that I shouldn't have been "had", that I ought to know better by now than to think I could simply go back and expect things to be as I left them. I didn't tell Diane how I felt, of course, because she made me very welcome, and the baby was sweet, but I knew that this would be my last trip to Lexby.

The second phone call was from Mum.

'Hi Mum.'

'I've got the news you've been waiting for. Ron and I and Jim and Sophie are having a joint wedding at Christmas!'

'That's wonderful. I haven't met Sophie yet. What's she like?'

'She's tall and slim and she's good for Jim – that's all that matters really. We're all invited to spend Christmas at Jim's new place in Coston, so you'll meet her then, if not before.'

I hadn't spoken to Max for nearly a year. In fact, whole weeks had passed without my even thinking about him. I used to go to Patrick's flat about once a fortnight after I'd left Arnold College, before he moved away, but recently, since everyone seemed to know I'd been in hospital, getting to see him meant running the risk of meeting groups of boys in the driveway. When they saw me coming, they would make noises they thought mad people made. Whoever had told them about me had obviously thought them mature enough to accept it; I just had to try and remember it wasn't their fault. I would probably have behaved in the same way at their age. In fact I know I would. I wondered how the subject had been introduced:

"Sir, has Miss Gates had a breakdown?" Perhaps this was in the middle of a fourth form lesson where I should have been, and where they were allowed to do their geography homework while a bored young maths teacher sat with them.

"As a matter of fact . . . Listen, all of you." Talking about it probably brightened up his day a bit. "You'll find out sooner or later anyway. Miss Gates *has* had a breakdown." There were sniggers I expect. "She was in hospital for a while, but I'm told she's much better now, although she won't be coming back. I hope I can rely on you to be sensible and not spread stupid rumours now you know the truth. It's an illness. We don't make fun of illnesses, now do we." Well, the way they heard it doesn't matter, but they weren't being very sensible or tactful when they saw me on my way to Patrick's.

'Gatters, can you pop to the offy to get a bottle of Fino?' He held out five pounds.

'Oh, Patrick, I don't want to go out again. Can't we make do with that bottle of red?'

'Oh, OK then.' He was surprised, but didn't ask why. And I was too embarrassed to give a reason.

When he left Arnold College, I knew I would never see him again. I felt it should have been I who was leaving first, because he was part of West Pluting and my memories of this school. Patrick moved up north to be nearer his ageing mother whom in the end he predeceased a few years later, at only fifty.

I went to his funeral, on a bleak November afternoon. It was two hundred and fifty miles from where I was now living. I sat staring at the coffin, decorated with a simple arrangement of white lilies. Strangers had gathered to say goodbye, their footsteps echoing on the stone floor of the dimly-lit chapel. The only man I recognised from Arnold College was the headmaster. We knelt to pray, each person wrapped in heavy coats and private memories. But I could not pray to a hostile God.

Patrick was taken back out to the hearse and tears stung my eyes. This was all there was. People filed out. I decided not to go on to the crematorium. Then I heard a voice behind me and turned round.

'Miss . . . Miss Gates?' A young woman with long dark hair was standing there, in a black coat. I hadn't been called Miss Gates in this way for a while.

'I'm sorry . . . do I know you?'

'It's Rachel, Miss. Rachel Mills. I was at Arnold College; you helped me.'

'Oh!'

She hugged me. We shared a taxi to the station, not daring to talk too much about the past. We left on separate trains.

My favourite place in West Pluting had always been the Topp. From the broad, high platform of grass and tarmac, with its row of flagpoles and memorials, you can look out over a vast expanse of ocean. There is a promontory each side like the wings of a theatre; on the stage at various times can be seen frigates, liners or speedboats scarring the surface of the water. Ships on the horizon look as if they staple together the sea and sky. On bad days, these were often the same colour. But this was a good day. The sun shot moving golden threads on the water and there was a stiff breeze which set the flags proudly declaring their allegiance and the ropes clanging against the poles.

It was more like July than September, the air like champagne. On days like this I liked to sit on one of the benches and watch people walking their dogs. It had been a good place to come when I was recovering. Today I had an appointment with Lucy in an hour, but I came here to collect my thoughts. I felt as though I was on holiday; my heart was with the flags.

Holidays. I hadn't had one for years, because it had been holiday OR car, right through my teaching career. The week before in West Pluting, things had changed. Then they'd changed again.

The first change was one to which I had given some thought and was now resigned. I'd thanked the middle-aged man and closed the door of number 79. He'd taken the documents and the car keys and driven off. Up to then, I had been concentrating on making a successful sale, deliberately ignoring how his visit and departure might affect me. Now it had come to this. I sat down and looked at the wad of £50 notes in my hand. The flat was silent. I felt suddenly deprived, grounded. I would have to get the train up to Howcester. But I knew that there was no getting round this decision: it was either car *or* rent this time. Nobody had told me if there was such a thing as Housing Benefit, but running a car was too expensive in any case.

Regarding the second change, I hoped it would be for the better. I was glad of Lucy's continuing support. She was the only person to whom I could talk freely about my situation, and over the months, I had been allowed to cry, laugh, even shout and scream, and I did. I knew every book spine in her office from avoiding eye-contact. Today, I would be more likely to laugh. I caught the bus up the hill from the town centre to the clinic.

'Come in, Vee.' She closed the door. 'Now, I've got your diary and – .'

'– Before you go any further, I've got some news for you.'

'Oh?' She put her hands in her lap and smiled.

'I've finally got a job! You know, the one I had the interview for a few days ago.'

'Congratulations! When do you start?'

'In three weeks' time. It's a place called the Squaremile Centre, for disabled people. I'm going to be a care assistant. It's not far from where my Mum lives, too.'

'That'll be very different for you. So that means we've only got one more session after today.'

'Actually, do you mind if this is our last meeting? Only there's a lot to do. Lucy, I just want to say thank you. I feel as if I've got my confidence back and my thoughts aren't so black any more. I remember how I used to think that I'd let the family down, because I wasn't perfect.'

'And what do you think now?' Her kind hazel eyes showed her pleasure.

'That nobody has to justify their existence by getting everything right. I also knew – in theory – that the kind of person you are is more important than what qualifications you have; that was my way of stopping myself from criticising other people. Now I'm trying really hard to put it into practice.'

'Good. That's important, Vee. Because accepting others and accepting yourself are actually the same thing.'

In the two years since Tor ward, I had seen the white door creak ajar once or twice, but it had closed again after a few days. In fact it blended in so well with its surroundings now, that its outline was scarcely visible on the healed surface.

Just because you know the way to your own private hell, it doesn't mean the devil's any less frightening. But the whole experience has a way of being dimmed by the passage of time, in the same way that you can't recall physical pain. But while this might be a relief, allowing you a period of time to enjoy yourself, it makes the next attack no less painful. Or predictable.

Curious to see if my memory of it matched the reality, I decided to pay a final visit to the hospital on the moor. I noticed that the bus service to the small village had been reduced. It was a bright, cold Saturday. I walked up the steep slope from the bus stop, past the whitewashed houses probably built to house the original "attendants". There was the H sign on its striped pole, bent over and green with algae.

I reached the entrance and gasped. Gone was Tor ward at the foot of the hill; in its place was a building site, an open wound, extending halfway up towards the clock tower of the old asylum, which I could just make out. It must be listed, I thought. To my left a large sign had been erected:

'Coming Soon! Luxury Retirement Apartments. For details, contact . . . ' The site resembled a familiar face whose teeth had been removed. As I turned away I felt a heavy disappointment. But why should I feel so attached to a place I had once dreaded, where I had lost control and which represented failure? And where were the cigarette men now?

When I got home, I rang Mum and told her about the hospital.

'Never mind. They seem to be doing that now across the country, then building new clinics as part of ordinary hospitals. Still, you're moving on now, anyway, aren't you? Your new job awaits. Exciting, isn't it? Ron and Jim say they'll be free that day to load up your stuff and bring it to Squaremile, with the trailer. Aren't you lucky – and to have got somewhere to live on site!'

'Yes. I don't know how I'd have managed.'

I arrived at the Squaremile Centre in October, not knowing anything at all about what my new job entailed. No details had been supplied at interview, so I naïvely thought I would just be spending time with the people there. The pay was less than I had been getting as a teacher, so there was no chance of replacing the car, but I had to seize any opportunity. I had told them I'd been depressed, but for once they didn't seem to mind.

I looked forward to making a fresh start here. The Centre was about three miles from the village of Whyton, on the top of a hill, so it was lucky I had accommodation on site, because an early shift started at 7.30, around the time of the first bus up from the village. There were six large residential houses, three on each side of the road which ran through the Centre. I would be working on Forest House. The others were called Birch, Sycamore, Orchard, Alder and Grove. All six houses were purpose-built when Squaremile was established in the early 1900s and they were regularly modernised. Each had a distinctive appearance and atmosphere, and was home to between fifteen and twenty-five residents. It had a Manager, a Deputy, sometimes a Subdeputy, a housekeeper and a team of staff, which included me. I was shocked to discover that we were the utter dogs' bodies.

Every morning the residents had to be got up, which in some cases meant using a hoist. It had to be recorded whether they were bathed, washed or showered, then, in this all-male house they were shaved, dressed and taken along to the dining room for breakfast. Some had calipers. Some needed to be fed.

It was hard physical work. On Forest, we would have three staff working with seventeen residents, to a deadline. The residents had to be ready to go to the Activities Unit for nine o'clock. They all had brain injuries of one kind or another, some had epilepsy and in Forest, which I soon realised was the heaviest house to work on, nearly all had varying degrees of physical disability as well. While the residents were out, we had to make the beds, changing sheets as necessary, wash the clothes, clean the bathrooms and keep the paperwork up to date, with the occasional meeting thrown in for good measure. Sometimes a resident had to be driven to a specialist appointment. But everything had to be done in time for when they were brought back for lunch.

The Activities Unit was situated at one end of the road, with the Day Hospital and admin. block at the other, making a huge rectangle. In amongst these buildings and the houses were therapeutic gardens, a chapel, kitchens, a repair shop, the laundry, a hall for concerts and, behind each of Forest, Grove, Birch, Sycamore, Orchard and Alder, a small number of staff flats: Old Oak to the east and New Beech to the west.

Old Oak was made up of four flats, two on each floor. Each flat was shared by two or three members of staff, but it was rare for anyone to live there longer than a few months: people either left completely or found somewhere else to live away from the Centre. There was a rapid turnover of junior staff.

By the entrance to Old Oak lived a middle-aged lady whom I hardly ever saw, with a cat called Phisto. His bed, food and water were always in the porch and when he got to know me he would be waiting for me when I came home, early or late, as if he had a copy of my duties and a watch. Sometimes he would come up to my flat on the first floor and sit by the radiator while I had a bath. He was very affectionate and I was delighted to be able to take him on when the lady downstairs left.

Sharing with complete strangers was something I hadn't done since my student days, but at least they didn't mind feeding Phisto if I went away for a couple of days. I did have to make sure my room was locked when I left for work and I had to know exactly what was in my section of the fridge. There was also competition for the bathroom, difficult if we were all on earlies.

I think I got off to a good start though, despite the unpleasant nature of some of the work. I don't think there is a single bodily fluid or function that I didn't encounter – or have to clean up – during the first month. My boss, Brendan Donnelly, RMN, was a good-natured, patient man and I learned a lot from him. There were protocols in care. For example, you had to be especially aware and tactful with some of the male residents, because the enforced intimacy, part of their everyday life, could lead to misunderstandings if they had never had a proper relationship. Indeed, very few had. All this was new ground to me: I had never shaved anyone before, let alone helped someone in the toilet.

Brendan soon saw that he could put my communication skills to good use on Forest. I was always the one he turned to for help with the wording of a notice or document, or if a meeting had to be organised. It was Centre policy that each resident have a "My Life" meeting annually, to which relatives and others involved with his or her care were formally invited. The resident's health, needs, activities, interests and future goals were examined and explored, the aim being to give him or her a sense of purpose, while at the same time reassuring visitors that we were doing our best for their family member. So I was frequently kept occupied with writing tasks in the afternoons. Brendan also trained me in giving out medication; although I was only a Second Grade, he knew I was more than capable. I was older than the other juniors, and he trusted me. If you are trusted, you feel confident.

The staff on the House were friendly enough, but here I had to make another adjustment, and get used to working alongside people who did not have the same educational history. Their common sense saw them through and they were quite content to live on the surface of life without feeling any need to look deeper. More importantly, they were happy with who they were. I knew I was a bit of a curiosity to begin with, but Brendan stamped out any hint of jealousy by saying that everybody had skills to bring to the workplace.

The trouble was, the junior staff saw writing as a soft option. If I was sitting preparing agendas or whatever, I wasn't working; for my workmates, only physical work was *real* work. For the first time in my life I had been made to feel guilty about writing. But I was learning a lot and I tried hard not to rock the boat, although I had to smile one day when a Starter Grade claimed she could not see to a resident straight away because she'd "only got two pairs of hands".

Overtime was available, on any house, but I found I could only manage two Long Days (7.30 a.m. to 9 p.m.) in a row on Forest, and that only if I had days off afterwards. Getting overtired was one factor in becoming unwell; I didn't want to find the white door open again. But I had to admit that I missed the adrenalin of the highs – before they went out of control, of course. The lithium and the other medication I was taking gave me a flatness which seemed to take the edge off daily experience. Rather this however, than go into the blackness again.

Preparing for Christmas with the residents was fun, even if it did mean taking them shopping for their own presents. Oh no, I wasn't thinking about bad things all the time, even if Aunt Mary lay dormant in my head. Part of my brain was always going to be her crypt, but it was well-concealed.

It was difficult to avoid becoming attached to some of the residents. I formed a special bond with one in particular: he was known as JD. This morning, typically, he had stated that he wanted to wear "long-sleeved socks, please". He'd had brain surgery at the age of twenty. Now forty, he could not walk unaided and his thinking was like a young child's. So taking him shopping could be tricky: if he saw something he wanted, the world had to know. Tantrums were sometimes unavoidable. I was his keyworker, which meant that other staff came to me if they were planning something which involved JD.

I managed to get Christmas Day and Boxing Day off, along with the week beforehand, as a special favour because of the wedding on 22nd. It meant I'd have to work New Year, but that didn't bother me.

Mum and I met up to choose our outfits at the end of November. Jim had told her that Sophie was expecting! A boy!

'You here Chrimmas, Vee?' JD's wheelchair had developed a squeak, I noticed.

'No, but I'll be back soon after.'

'Ow. Where goin'?'

'To see my family.'

'Where they live, then?'

'Oh, not far away.'

''Cos I got a prezzie for you. I love you, Vee!'

15

Porteblanche

I don't remember much about that Christmas, even now. ECT does that, taking out whole swathes. The double wedding took place, but it was now a blur, blotted out by the malicious spring which followed.

I recall how everything was all too green and urgent again, with the exam bird singing for its life. Brendan seemed worried. The juniors on Forest were looking at me, then pulling faces at each other. I didn't know why: I felt fine, full of energy and working at top speed. Then the white door opened and I plunged into the trap, the black tunnel, with its rows of slamming train doors. I crashed.

'Vee?' I could see Brendan's arms on the dining table. 'I think you should go home. Did you know that you've been high as a kite all morning?'

I couldn't answer. I deserved to fail again. Back at Old Oak, Phisto curled up on the bed next to me, purring his comfort. I'd put on a manic display I didn't recall and I felt guilty and embarrassed, so I couldn't cry. I don't know how long I was lying there, or who came and found me, or what they did, but I remember being helped into an ambulance by people who smelt faintly of iodine and clean, whole, other lives. Perhaps I was going to the moor.

When I returned to my much thinner body after what seemed like weeks of endless night, a nurse was sitting by my bed. 'Vee? Oh good. You're back. You had us all worried!'

'Where..?' I coughed. My mouth was not used to speaking. 'Where am I?' I whispered.

'In the Porteblanche Unit at Howcester General. Are you thirsty? Hungry?'

'Water, please,' I managed, drank, then fell asleep. A rough sea of moods had thrown me around for what seemed like an age, until the extra drugs and ECT began to take effect and calm the waves. I would be right up there with the lightning, then I would crash into the depths. Eventually I would be washed ashore and able to see the highs and lows as separate from me, the changes in the tide as less threatening, the black clouds fading. It became a familiar pattern. For the time being, however, there was Freda.

'Why did you let yourself get into that dreadful state?' she asked angrily, as if I had deliberately wasted her time and NHS resources. I realised that Freda thought I had not been taking my medication, but I could not find the words to defend myself.

Whether you were very ill or recovering, a good nurse would talk to you the same way. Your validity as a human being would not be in doubt. Such nurses represented stability; they were reference points for normality, coming in from their own separate, normal lives. They didn't mock, they had compassion, discretion and best of all, they listened. I'd met plenty of them in Tor ward.

But nowadays, here in this Porteblanche place, talking to patients was out of fashion for nurses, it seemed. Nor did it matter any more, apparently, if they expressed negative opinions or made assumptions about people in their care when those people were present, or spoke about them in a derogatory way as if the patients were deaf. These so-called nurses were like schoolchildren trying to impress their friends. Some of them, including Freda, were no better at being a nurse than someone brought in from the street.

Had the training changed, the emphasis? The attempts to understand, the time spent listening, were scarce. There was nobody here like Ian from Tor ward, in whom I could confide or to whom I could express my anxiety. Most of the nurses just sat in the office chatting and laughing until late when we were trying to sleep. They were merely onlookers, reluctant to help, quick to find fault, except for a few. My brain had closed off and now I was closed off from the staff – from nearly everyone, in fact.

I felt desperate. Oh, I couldn't take another day inside this head which I couldn't control, and I had to do something about it. So I started to plan. I confided in another patient. I was lying on my bed when Freda marched in without knocking.

'Got your affairs in order then, have you?' she asked with venom. 'Let me tell you something.' She put her face to within two feet of mine. 'If you attempt suicide, you will be moved to the Secure Unit. In there, you'll have no visitors and no ECT. Think about it.'

She removed all the coathangers from my wardrobe, then swept out of the room without another word. When I thought about this, I realised she'd not only come across as menacing, but she'd lied! Of course people in the Unit got visitors and ECT! Why would she say that? In a world where I wasn't wanted or needed, which would no doubt be relieved when I wasn't around any more, where the smallest dot of interference from me in other people's normality was unacceptable, there was something I couldn't understand: how could doing something so right for me, so right for the world, produce such a hostile reaction in someone considered normal?

In Tor ward you had been allowed to smoke anywhere except in your bedroom, but here they had a designated smoking room, a sign of the times. I could envisage a future where there would be no smoking room at all and patients (and staff) would have to go somewhere outside, because the staff here hated having to enter the smoking room. I could understand that – it did get a bit thick in there sometimes.

But for now, Porteblanche smoking room was the centre of the universe. You could listen to music, chat, or just sit and smoke. In the corner was a large man with a mountain of long black hair. He would remain quite still for a long while with his hair forward, completely concealing his face. Then he would suddenly fling the hair back and sit up straight, like a whale surfacing for air. A black woman paced up and down, talking loudly to an invisible friend about life on the street. From time to time she alarmed everyone by launching into a stream of abuse at top volume.

As my mood swings grew less dramatic, I became aware of a curious ward hierarchy: the two young men who always wore the same clothes were drug addicts, the lowest form of life on the ward according to the patients I spoke to. They only had one thing on their mind: to get out. Once or twice they went missing for a day, but were brought back. Then came the schizophrenics, who didn't really understand what was going on a lot of the time. Top of the tree were those of us no longer referred to as manic depressive, but as "bipolar". The alcoholics, amost as lowly as the drug addicts, would try and mimic the bipolars to score points and get attention from the nurses. But we could see through them. Oddly enough, being bipolar was apparently a desirable state. With the name change from manic depression, who knows? Perhaps "being bipolar" would catch on as a fashion accessory like a chihuahua under the arm, for people who would never have a clue about its true nature. It would be like believing you could befriend a hurricane.

I had eight treatments. We could sit outside in the garden if we were well enough and I noticed that roses were in bloom. Mum arrived.

'Oh, you're looking much better than when I last came, Vee!' She had tears in her eyes. 'I've brought you some bits and pieces. Has Jim been, or phoned the ward?'

'I don't know, Mum. I'm only just beginning to make sense of this.'

'Only they've got some news. I don't suppose they'll mind me telling you but Matthew was born last night in the hospital here, next door. All's well apparently. I expect Jim will be in touch.' She was obviously very proud. 'Have you seen a psychiatrist yet?'

'I'm due to see one tomorrow.'

I was an aunt!

The next morning Freda was on. I always knew when handover was finished because there would be a sudden burst of voices when the office door opened. I heard Freda's voice and strange little laugh.

Eventually it was time for the ward round.

Max had not observed life on a psychiatric ward from the same perspective as Vee of course. Helen was glad he had Vee's book to occupy his time; she was very busy at work, and he was left to his own devices for most of the day. He had caught up with Helen now, and reading kept Vee's memory alive for him, to such an extent that he thought he could sometimes feel emotions from her, as if she were in the attic room with him. So he read on. Ah, yes. Vee was about to be called into the ward round. He wished it could have been different.

'Dr Greenwood will see you now, Vee. Through here.' She smiled. It was a kind nurse who had spoken to me before. Dr Greenwood? My heart . . .

I knew I would have to put my face straight quickly and hide my surprise, pretend not to know him. I was well enough, and I had been in the system long enough, to grasp that. There wasn't time to think about anything else.

I was shown into the small room reserved for ward rounds at the end of a corridor. Max sat under the window, facing me as I came in, with a nurse on each side. He had a folder in his lap.

'Hello, Vee. Do take a seat.' His voice was controlled but gentle. The look he gave me, though brief, conveyed the message: "yes, it's me, but you don't know me, OK?" Just as I'd predicted. He was ten years older of course, his hair had receded and was now completely grey, but it was definitely Max.

'How are you feeling now, after ECT? You've been in quite a bad way.'

'Much better thank you,' I replied.

'Would you like to go on weekend leave tomorrow? Then if all goes well, we can think about discharging you next week. But I would like to arrange for you to see a CPN – that's a Community Psychiatric Nurse – when you're back at home. Anything you want to ask me?'

That was cruel! Of course there were things I wanted to ask him! He opened the folder briefly. Then his steady gaze, over his reading glasses, and his mask of professional detachment left me in no doubt as to how to respond.

'No. I . . . I'll go for the weekend leave, please.'

He was lucky: *he'd* had time to get used to the idea of meeting me! Come to think of it, he must have seen me at my worst without my knowledge. A host of memories suddenly mingled with the embarrassment of my present situation and refused to be submerged: Max undoing my blouse . . . caressing and kissing . . . It wasn't supposed to be like *this!* I wasn't supposed to be his *patient!* The knowledge that I had done what was necessary for the time being was my only consolation.

On the weekend leave, I went shopping with Mum. I had a warm welcome from Phisto at the flat, but a silent reception from one of the girls I shared with. I think it had something to do with my resemblance to an axe-murderer. I attacked the pile of post waiting for me. When finally I returned to Old Oak properly, there was one more letter to open. Personnel had sent it through the internal mail: they wanted me to attend a disciplinary hearing.

'Why . . . why cryin', Vee?' JD caught sight of me when I arrived at Forest House two days after coming out of Porteblanche.

'I'm OK, JD.'

'Not OK. Here . . . here . . . ' He was holding out his arms for a hug, but I decided against it as he had spilt breakfast down his front.

'I'll see you later, right? You should be at Activities, shouldn't you?'

'OK. S'pose so.'

I wanted to talk to Brendan, who came out of the office just at that moment.

'Vee cryin', Brendan.' JD had followed me in his wheelchair and was worried.

'Oh, hello. Were you after me?' Brendan showed every sign of being busy.

'I've had a letter I'd like you to look at.'

'Go and sit in there. I'll be back in a minute.' I waited, looking absently at the notices which had appeared during my time off. Brendan came back and shut the door.

'Now, let's see.' He read the letter standing up. At more than six feet, he towered over me. 'Oh, so the hearing's in . . . half an hour. The trouble is, Vee, they see an absence like this as you failing in terms of performance, which is all that matters to them.'

'But when I'm well, I do a reasonable job, don't I?'

'Wh . . . yes, you do! Better than reasonable. But absence means you don't, if you see what I mean. It kind of . . . cancels it out.' The phone rang. 'I'll ring you back', he muttered hastily into it. 'Vee, they can't tell the difference between a bad performance at work and not being at work at all. That's what you're up against. Their policies don't cover your circumstances.'

'So what do I do?'

'You go to the meeting and stick up for yourself. That's all you can do. I can't really help beyond that, I'm afraid. They've seen the good reports I've written about you. I take it a Union rep will be there to support you?'

'Yes. I met up with him yesterday afternoon. It was the first thing I did after opening the letter. It's Bernie from the repair shop. I don't know if he'll be any use, quite honestly. I don't think he really grasped what was happening.'

'Well, I wish you luck. By the way,' he added, with a friendly smile, 'It's good to see you looking much better than when I saw you in Porteblanche.' He turned and picked up the phone. So he'd visited me! I wished I could remember. And who else had? It was a disturbing idea. And I had to admit that, although I had told them at interview that I'd been depressed, I don't think anyone, including me, had anticipated a three-month spell in hospital. Was the medication wrong? Oh, I had so much to ask Max! What made things worse at this stage was that I was still trying to find the real me again, so I wasn't as strong as I'd have liked going into this hearing. The white door wasn't quite shut, but I was treated as if it was; most people, after all, only have one state of being, and are fortunate not to know other mental dimensions.

'Come in, sit down.' Susan Perry, the Personnel Manager, sounded weary and distant. She was a pale-faced woman of about my age who spoke with a Yorkshire accent and always wore a short skirt and jacket. There were two men in suits in the office as well.

'You've met Jack Marshall and Tim Clark, Senior Managers, haven't you Miss Gates? You will appreciate,' she went on, without giving me a chance to reply, 'that absences of this length cannot be tolerated. They put a great strain on us in terms of manpower.' Her voice sounded mechanical.

'I do realise that, yes, but I couldn't help it.'

'Now . . . we know you've had problems, but you see, if everyone took three months off when they felt like it, we'd be in a right mess. Think about it. And think about your colleagues for once.' This was said with emphasis, so that I felt like a naughty child. But I had to speak up, take Brendan's advice, as Bernie didn't seem able to take part.

'I was actually ill in hospital. It wasn't that I felt like taking time off!'

Ms Perry showed all the understanding of which she was capable, which meant ignoring what I had to say. 'Be that as it may, the result's the same for the Centre. And if you were in hospital, Miss Gates, how do you account for the fact that you were seen at your flat a few days ago?' It was obvious she held all the cards.

'I was on weekend leave. That's what they do, to see if you're ready to come out of hospital.' As expected, this had no effect.

'We have decided to give you a verbal warning at this stage.' She glanced at a folder on her desk. 'According to our records, you have only worked for seventy-five per cent of your time here. That's not good enough.' She paused. Brendan was right. Then came a bizarre question. 'When are you going to be ill again?'

A groan of disbelief was all Bernie could manage. I couldn't believe it either. It was like asking someone when they would next catch cold.

'I don't know.' This was all I dared answer, because in a split second, I suspected that the question was designed to provoke me. An angry outburst wouldn't help my cause at all.

I left the department feeling sick and bad-tempered. There was guilt, too, introduced by Ms Perry's overriding concern with staff numbers. I could have done without that, and their suspicions; I was still struggling to get my life back together, and it was clear I was on my own.

16

Cakes, Sophie and Max

ECT does not discriminate between short-term and long-term memory. If a plate of cakes represents the mind, ECT is the hand which can take memories at random from any part without your knowledge. Some of the cakes reappear at different times, and some take longer to find their cue. But some disappear for ever. So it was with the Christmas before Porteblanche. I have a vague memory of the wedding, however, which went something like this.

I remember knowing it was hard for me to join in with the excitement all around me. I only really caught a little of the atmosphere in that small room, when the registrar, a short woman in an embroidered suit, began her important and dignified address. Even then, I watched as if I were an observer from another world.

' . . . Pamela and Ronald . . . and James and Sophie . . . before these witnesses . . . Pamela and Ronald first, please . . . '

Mum was wearing a fitted cream dress and short-sleeved jacket ("We won't bother with hats!"). She carried a simple mixed bouquet. Ron wore a pale grey suit, waistcoat and bright blue tie. As they stood together, from my seat in the front row I could see the edge of Mum's jacket quivering. Her voice was thin and higher-pitched than usual, but I knew she meant every word.

There were Christmas swags along the seats. Vows and rings were exchanged, and when the cheers and applause had died down, the registrar called Jim and Sophie forward. Jim also had on a smart light grey suit and slightly darker tie, with a very pale blue shirt. Sophie was in a frothy, low-cut white creation. Her parents were clearly moved. Outside, bouquets and confetti were thrown and a cheer went up when one of the bridesmaids caught Sophie's flowers. All the usual stuff that happens. As for the reception, it is a complete blank apart from the amazing cake. It's a shame, I know, and I've probably imagined a lot of this to compensate for what has been lost. Sometimes it's hard to tell the difference.

Nevertheless, that old feeling was with me throughout: weddings were not part of my life and never would be. These people, however close they were to me, were separated from me by an invisible divide. It wasn't that I didn't love them: I just couldn't share their joy.

Whether the memory was accurate or not, what I *feel* has no connection with ECT or illness. It was normal for me to think that I could never hope to cross into the world which *real* people took for granted. Something was missing in me: love was too difficult, too complicated, so how could I ever get married? It was out of the question. I knew I would always be alone.

The feeling of alienation was compounded by a sense of not being on the same wavelength as Sophie. I couldn't remember if we'd had a disagreement, or what it was exactly. I couldn't pin it down, but there was definitely something not right. As for her relationship with Jim, it was none of my business, so I kept my thoughts to myself. I was hardly in a position to judge her, and if Jim was happy, which he obviously was, then I had to accept his new wife.

I had a text from Jim a few days after the nightmare hearing, suggesting we meet up. No more "memory cakes" of the Christmas wedding had resurfaced, but I had to pretend they had. I was looking forward to seeing my nephew for the first time.

We found a corner of the pub which wasn't too noisy. Matthew was in a buggy, crying. He stopped briefly when I said hello, but then carried on; I laughed. Sophie got a bottle out for him and picked him up. The Lion, in Howcester, was where Jim said he came sometimes before he went to university. Sophie was quiet, appearing a little on edge.

Jim returned with our drinks. 'What's it like being back at work then, Vee?' he asked.

'Oh, you know. Still getting used to it. But I've got a new ally now, a CPN.' Jim knew what that meant of course, but spelt it out for Sophie's benefit. 'Her name is Bella and she came to see me for the first time yesterday. She seems nice.'

'That's good. You could do with some support, from what you've told me.'

Still Sophie remained silent.

'Yes. She was horrified to hear that I'd been disciplined for something I can't help. In fact, it's strange, but I hadn't realised that this hearing was anything out of the ordinary. I'd just accepted it, until I saw Bella's reaction. It reminded me of telling Mum the price of something and hearing her say, "*How* much?!"'

Jim smiled. Sophie sipped her drink.

'So Bella will be keeping an eye on you. But Vee – you might never be ill again!'

'Maybe, but I've read that if you've had more than one episode, it's likely it'll happen again. Apparently it's a combination of genetics and a severe stress which starts the illness off, after which it develops a timetable, a momentum of its own, regardless of stress. And even if you take your tablets.'

At last Sophie spoke. 'Isn't it all just an attitude of mind, though?'

'What do you mean?' I had forgotten the way I used to think, but now I was looking at it again, this time like a cast-off skin.

'I mean, this "*illness*". Pha, we all get depressed, after all. You just have to get through it. Take today, for instance. Someone scratched my car, and I was really fed up. But I didn't let it ruin my life! You have to be a bit tougher, Vee. And as for tablets, well . . . '

I felt a hot surge of anger in my stomach. 'Oh, really?' was all I could manage, with false cheer and a sudden desire to walk out. Jim could tell that things were getting awkward and opted for a diversion.

'Oh, look!' he said, pointing to a noisy gathering. 'They're obviously having their reception here. Brings back memories.' He kissed Sophie on the cheek.

I composed myself. I had to concentrate on the fact that she was *lucky* not to understand. Her skies were a cloudless blue. Once, a long time ago, I had believed I was invincible too. There was a pause for ruffled feathers to subside and put themselves straight, but I suddenly felt as if only two or three people in the whole world could help me, and I longed to see Max again.

I tried not to think about Sophie too often over the next few days; her comments raised my blood pressure and I would find it hard to get off to sleep.

It was my first day back full-time. On Forest House the routine hadn't changed, but I had to re-learn certain things eroded or erased by ECT. Sometimes memories – "cakes"– returned without any effort on my part. This might occur quite spontaneously in the course of a conversation, or while doing some ordinary task.

But at other times, no matter how hard I tried to conceal it, there would be embarrassment. Nobody knows how many memories they have, so I had no way of telling which ones were missing. Seen another way, finding memories stolen by ECT was like blundering about in the dark and stumbling upon familiar pieces of furniture.

'Is tea ready yet, Vee?' JD asked.

'No, er . . . can you lay the tables for me please. I think it's your turn.'

'OK. Then you get tea, yeah?'

'Are you hungry?' I asked, smiling but wondering how I was supposed to conjure up this meal.

'Yeah.'

'So'm I,' said John, another resident. And now even those who couldn't speak were getting agitated as well. I was beginning to panic. Where was the tea? Did I have to cook it myself, and with what? Brendan came into the kitchen. 'Everything OK?' he asked, his tone of voice letting me know he was worried.

'Fine, except that I don't seem to have anything for their tea.'

Brendan looked at me with ill-concealed surprise. 'The trolley will be here in a few minutes. I've just sent Mags over to collect it.' He said this as calmly as he could. Suddenly I felt stupid as this memory cake crashed down so hard it almost broke the plate. I was so ashamed I ran off to the toilet. Of course the hot trolley would come from the kitchens! It was usually small details which came back, but this was a major disaster, a memory lapse of such magnitude that, despite Brendan's reassurance, I did not recover my equanimity for some while. The residents were oblivious, which made things a little easier, but I couldn't help asking myself if there might be another crash soon. And once again I was alone in this experience. Oh, Max.

I arrived at the hospital in a thunderstorm for our next appointment. When the bus pulled up at the request stop at the far end of Howcester General, everyone on board knew you were going to Porteblanche. Oh well.

After a short while, my name was called. The double doors buzzed as the receptionist let me through. Just before the offices, to the right, a flight of stairs plunged down and round a corner to the lower floor, where the acute wards were situated, out of sight. I had gone down those steps only months beforehand, in an altered state of mind. Painful memories had to be shut down as I passed. The smell of the place, too, a mixture of stale tobacco and cleaning fluid, brought back the feeling of being "in" again, or "on the farm" as some people called it. All the doors were stiff and creaked, echoing in the corridor. I approached the row of offices, my footsteps now muffled by a carpet whose pattern I recognised from the ward, although it was a different shade and much cleaner. I had seen it when I came up to this floor for ECT. The last room bore his name. I knocked.

'Come in!' Max got to his feet. We stood for a moment, not knowing what to do. Then, resisting the urge to throw myself forward and embrace him, I sat down. 'How are you, Vee?' It was that quiet, gentle voice which I had tried so hard to forget. He sat in the other armchair and crossed his legs.

'Fine.' I didn't know where to start. 'I thought you were in Edinburgh.' For a second, I felt deceived.

'I was, but . . . well, a lot's happened since then.' He straightened his jacket. 'When I saw your name on one of the files, I was . . . surprised. I mean I knew you'd been a bit down when we spoke on the phone, but – .'

'– How d'you think I felt when I walked into that ward round?!' A burst of indignation got the better of me. 'I'd only just heard your name, for God's sake!'

'I'm really sorry about that, Vee, believe me. It wasn't very fair. But I couldn't see any other way. As you gathered – and I knew you would – if either of us had revealed that we knew one another, I would've had to pass your case on to a colleague. And I wanted to – .'

'– Is that all I am now, just a "case"?'

'No, Vee. That's the point! I wanted to see you again and talk to you, and I wouldn't have been able to if – .'

'– Why didn't I get to see you before that, though?'

'Because you were too ill. I was there . . . I saw you, but you might have blurted something out if you'd seen me. It would have been hard to explain to others.' He rubbed his forehead.

'Supposing I'd *wanted* to see another doctor? Had you thought of *that*?' I slammed my fist down on the arm of the chair. We sat in silence for a moment, while the rain rattled on the window.

'Look, you can if you . . . ' He sighed. 'I can understand your embarrassment, Vee, but you have to believe me when I say that I don't think any less of you. There is . . . one thing I should mention though. Something important.' I could see the anxiety in his eyes. I struggled to calm down.

'What is it, Max? I can still call you that, at least, can't I?'

'Of course – in here.' He grimaced. 'Vee, I'm . . . married now with two young daughters.'

It was not as painful as I'd feared, but I had to strengthen my voice as I remembered our lost baby. I couldn't tell him now. Something, a knot somewhere, untied itself because it needed to be free, to escape for ever.

'The nearest I've got is becoming an aunt. Yes, Jim's a dad now.'

'Oh, pass on my congratulations, won't you.' Max smiled.

'So, where did you meet your wife?'

'In Edinburgh. She's a nurse. I know! Corny, isn't it, doctors and nurses!' He was trying to lighten the atmosphere.

'And how old are your daughters?' I smiled politely.

'Grace is nine and Anna is nearly eight. Vee, I'm still here to help you, but I had to tell you that in case – .'

'– It's OK, Max. I understand. I know that this is a doctor's appointment and nothing else. But there is one thing you haven't told me yet, and that's why you came back down here.'

'My parents lived a few miles from here and my father became very ill. My mother couldn't look after him. I was lucky to get this job. With consultant posts, it's very often a case of waiting for dead men's shoes, but Porteblanche was a new department. Then dad died and I had to make arrangements for mum to be looked after, until she died the following year.'

'Thank you for telling me, Max. Now I want . . . I think we need to close off our private lives. Unless you want to ask me anything.'

He had been leaning forward for a while. Now he sat back and crossed his ankles. 'OK, Vee. Shall we spend a few minutes looking at how things are for you these days? Bella's filled me in on how difficult work's been. I think it's outrageous that you should have been put through a disciplinary hearing. Outrageous. Anyway, how are your moods?'

'OK. The memory blanks are the big thing. But I still get

the occasional "up" swing. That's when I write my best stuff.'

'Really? I didn't know you wrote! How come you kept such a big secret from me? What are you working on at the moment?'

'Max, I thought we'd separated off *now* from *then*. Please don't make it more difficult than it already is for me to see you as my doctor!'

'Sorry. Even trained psychiatrists get things wrong, you know.' He uncrossed his ankles and, his elbow on the arm of his chair, rested his chin in his hand, looking at me intently. 'Go on.'

'I write mostly poetry. If I'm high, poems can burst out of me, ready made, on to the paper. I can write when I'm OK, too. It's a good way of escaping, but it doesn't have quite the same magical quality as when I'm high.'

'I'm glad you're not high – or low – at the moment anyway. Look, this isn't necessarily connected with what you've just said, but our time is running out and I want to make some adjustments to your medication.' He stood up for a moment and reached for my file on a shelf. Then I listened as he instructed me in the dose change of one type of tablet, the stopping of another and the introduction of a new one. 'Anything else you want to talk about while you're here? You seem to be coping quite well.'

'I'll be alright.'

'So, shall we meet in three months' time? No, it'll have to be at the end of August, I think. Yes, because I'm away for part of September. Then if everything's OK, we can make it a six-monthly appointment.'

In the ten years that I worked at the Squaremile Centre, I had to go into hospital five times. Actually it was six, if I count the operation on my feet. Diane and Jeff got married during my third spell, as I found out too late, and Granny Wheeler died during the fourth. Something of significance to me or my family always seemed to happen when I was not able to participate.

Concerning my feet, time off for an operation was regarded as *proper* sick leave, so there was no disciplinary hearing or warning. What a difference it makes when you can *see* something's wrong; that must be the criterion for acceptable incapacity.

Mr Montgomery, the Chief Executive of Squaremile for the last twenty years, was present at my fourth hearing. He admitted that "disciplinary" was probably an inappropriate label for these hearings when they related to ill-health. A bit late, I thought. Whatever the title of the meeting, though, it didn't stop them from giving me a first and final written warning. I couldn't understand how I was supposed to heed the warnings and improve; the whole warnings process implied that my illness was as much under my control as a conscious act.

Monty, as he was known – though with what affection I hadn't a clue – had scarcely looked at me directly at that last hearing. When he did, his eyes seemed clouded with boredom. It was just another rubber stamp to him. But what use were warnings now? All they did was add official disapproval to something I didn't much like anyway. And the worst of it was, I could be out of the door if there was even the slightest suspicion I had made a mistake at work.

Then came terrible news. Mum rang me in tears to say that Sophie had died in a car accident. I rang Jim but there was no answer at home or on his mobile. Mum told me later that she and Ron had driven to Coston to be with him and little Matthew, who couldn't understand where Mummy had gone. I remembered Dad.

Sophie had been expecting a baby sister for Matthew. After a few days, I spoke to Jim, but I didn't know how to console him.

17

Promotion

I had been at Forest House for seven years, and was frequently left as "senior-on", as they called it, when there was nobody else to take charge. Although I was in Squaremile's bad books, with all the hearings and warnings, I was still expected to run a house when it suited them, even as a mere Second Grade. I had to be reliable when they needed me; I suppose they thought I'd be too flattered to mind that no extra money came with the responsibility.

I began to think it was high time I tried to get the pay I'd been missing out on. Young girls with no qualifications were being promoted over me when they had been there two years or less. After a couple of attempts, my luck changed. There was a vacancy for a Sub-Deputy in Birch House. JD wheeled himself over to me.

'Why goin', Vee?'

'I've been promoted. It's good!'

'Not good for me. Don't go!'

I crouched down and looked at him. There were tears in his eyes. I put my hand on his shoulder. I told him I wasn't going far and that I'd still come and visit him, and do overtime shifts there.

'Oh? When?'

'I don't know yet, but I'll try to come as often as I can.'

'OK.' JD sped off howling, in search of a tissue, nearly colliding with another resident.

It was a relatively recent condition that you had to be a qualified nurse to run a house, so at this time there were still managers who had not done the training. Bill, the manager on Birch, was one example. When the time came for him to retire, he would be replaced by a nurse. Brendan had painted a grim picture of Bill, formerly a plumber, and it wasn't long before I found out why I had been the only one to apply for the post on Birch.

I wanted promotion so badly that I ignored the lack of competition for the job, just as I ignored Brendan's warnings. I wanted to prove that I could cope with more responsibility, while proving to myself that being bipolar did not diminish my ability. I had been patient. Now I wanted some action. I soon discovered, however, that my optimism and ideas got Bill's back up. He wanted to sail quietly into retirement, but then I came along to rock the boat. I had not set out to change his little world, just to do my best, but after two weeks of mounting tension, Bill exploded.

'Why did you put this up on the board?' he fumed, closing the office door sharply and waving my notice about laundry procedure in the air.

'People were putting things in the wrong colour bags,' I answered, honestly. Bill sat behind his desk, but I had a feeling he would not be there long.

'For one thing, I don't believe you and for another, couldn't you just have *told* them? You didn't need a notice!' The temperature was rising; an outburst was imminent.

'Yes, but it seemed easier, as I don't see everyone on every shift.'

'And what's this?' His anger reached boiling point. He was red in the face and stood up suddenly, large and threatening, pushing the chair away behind him with his legs. He was referring to a note I had left myself; he had assumed it was for him because I'd left it in the wrong place. The brevity of the note had made him jump to the wrong conclusion. I tried to explain, but by now he was in full flow.

'You have no respect for me!' he bellowed. 'I should never have agreed to your coming here. You come in, with your degree and your fancy ideas, trying to take over the place!

Never mind what *I've* done to get this house to where it is now!'

The thunder rolled on and I resigned myself to not getting a word in. I felt sick. Bill was not going to listen to anything I had to say anyway. He was the House Manager and woe betide anyone who challenged a single one of his decisions or procedures. When the storm was over, I opened the office door calmly, to find two junior staff looking rather sheepish. I did not make eye contact.

There was one faintly amusing aspect of Bill's behaviour, however: about a week after he'd dismissed one of my ideas out of hand, *he* would think of it, so that it became acceptable – good, even, something to point out and be praised for, when senior management came to call.

Pride is a strange thing if it is at another's expense. So is jealousy of someone with bipolar disorder, when you don't know the first thing about it. Normally jealousy, which can never hide for long, strives to make someone feel ashamed of something they would usually be proud of. In this case, fear was mixed with it. Bill had made this plain. He really didn't know what to make of me but at the same time he obviously felt threatened. I was better educated, but I was also a woman, and in his little world, Birch House, I should know my place. But then there was this strange illness; what might she do?

My reaction to this was to stay as calm and distant as possible; I had nothing to prove. This change of tactics however made Bill suspicious of my sudden desire to be part of the furniture and he began to push a bit, do things which he knew would annoy me. It was as if he *needed* an adversary. For instance, he kept giving me only two days off after a ten-day stretch, changing the rota in very bad grace when I pointed out, quietly, that this wasn't fair.

I was relieved that the situation was in the end short-lived. I was in sole charge one day and was expected to make a decision – I can't even remember what about now – but it was quite important at the time. Needless to say, it was the wrong decision for Bill when he came back. There was a showdown with senior management, my quiet protestations carried no weight and I was moved promptly to Alder House as an extra to be observed, under threat of demotion if I "caused any further problems".

Alder House residents were female and over fifty. Age did not, however, prevent them from being very much more vocal than their male counterparts about whether or not they should have a bath and what they should wear.

The House Manager was a woman called Sandra, who looked two or three years older than me, with short fair hair and darting brown eyes. Jean, her deputy, who agreed with everything Sandra said, was about sixty with a grown-up family. Sandra had no children, and seemed bitter about this. In normal mode (and she had several modes), there was a certain cynicism which tainted her dealings with others; the attitude of the House Manager is crucial and she had no idea that the way she coped with her own circumstances could have a significant effect on those she worked with. That was normal mode. I experienced others as time went by.

I knew that neither Sandra nor Jean wanted me on Alder House. I had been dumped on them, after all. The feeling of reluctant acceptance trickled down into the lower grades. Sandra seemed uneasy in my presence. I didn't know whether this was because she knew about my qualifications or because of the axe-murderer syndrome, but on the Centre, both were considered afflictions to be whispered about in corners. I don't think Sandra knew how to behave towards me, any more than Bill had, so she opted for the dismissive approach. I was a lower form of life.

'Vee, go and get the post now. Why haven't you thought to get it already?' It was raining. 'Nat, would you check through this list of supplies with me?'

Natalie, or Nat, as everyone called her, was a Starter Grade of about nineteen, but was obviously held in high regard. The post was collected twice daily from the admin block; it wasn't far, but still not pleasant in the rain. I took a carrier bag as I anticipated sarky comments about the letters being wet. She knew I couldn't refuse to go, but it wasn't the first time she'd made sure Nat, Sally or Liz had the "dry" jobs and sent me out. I got back to Alder just as Jack Marshall, Senior Manager, Care, arrived. I hadn't seen him much until then, apart from at my hearings, but I noticed he was becoming a regular visitor to the house.

'Do come in, Jack!' gushed Sandra. (Attempt at "light and feminine" mode?)

'Thank you. Not a nice day. Where can I put this?' He held out a dripping umbrella.

'Let me take it for you. There.' She put it in a stand by the door. 'Come through to the office. How are you? And Mrs Marshall?'

'We're fine, thank you. And you?'

'Fine, fine. Oh, don't sit there. Have this chair – it's more comfortable. What can I do for you?'

'Er, I wonder if we could have a word in private.'

'Sure. Vee, would you please go and see if tea's arrived yet love?' Another of Sandra's modes was being a good actress. I was glad to be able to leave the room.

As usual, I had nobody to talk to about these things except Bella. I got on with my work, but without the warmth of sharing jokes or stories from the past, which had brightened the day in Forest House. Doing the occasional shift in the old House was like putting on comfortable clothing after a day in something too tight. In Alder, by contrast, I had to apply what I had learned with Bill on Birch House; in other words I had to keep quiet and not voice an opinion about anything, as I knew that every word I said would get back to Sandra and be ripe for misinterpretation. There had always been something about me which seemed to invite criticism; though I couldn't understand why this was, I had to be alert at all times.

Sandra spent most of her shift chatting in the office: her territory. I would go in there only if absolutely necessary or if Jean was in charge. My permanent insanity gave Alder

House staff a comfortable ride. That sounds like a contra-
diction, but what I mean is that it afforded them the luxury
of being the responsible, level-headed ones, who were
always right. So if anything went wrong, it was easy to see
who would get the blame.

Catherine was one of only two residents on Alder who
smoked and along with Jean had to stand outside in the
porch when she wanted a cigarette. All three had terrible
coughs. An autumnal chill made the porch a draughty place.

'Bloody Norah, I could do with a brew!' Catherine
muttered as she came in, passing the office door, coughing
and rubbing her hands.

'I'm just going to put the kettles on,' I called. I liked
Catherine. She'd had a hard life according to the notes, but
she was always cheerful. She was sixty-six and very wrin-
kled, as if her brown paper face had been screwed up and
then flattened out again; her top lip looked as though it had
been blanket-stitched. Then there was June, in her late fifties,
who enjoyed helping me in the kitchen when she could.

'D'you know, Vee,' said June in her tiny voice, 'this is my
favourite weather today, cold and bright.' She put some
mugs on the tea trolley.

'I know, June. Oh, I meant to ask you: would you like to
go shopping next week? We could get you a new dress for
Christmas. Sandra said it would be OK.'

'That'd be lovely!'

I couldn't find any other staff on the house to help give
everyone their tea; they could have been toileting or fetch-
ing people from Activities, I reasoned, as it was about half
past three. I wasn't too concerned. June and I managed; at
least it made her feel she was doing something important,
I think. About half an hour after the ladies had had their
drinks, most of them had congregated in the lounge to
watch a particular programme. I took a couple of them to
the toilet, checked some of their rooms, then headed for the
office, where I had some phone calls to make before my
shift ended. The only sounds were the television and the
residents' laughter in response to it. I remembered there

was also some urgent paperwork after my calls. The office was quiet. But where were Sandra and Nat? It seemed I had been left on my own, just when I was due off. A knock at the open door startled me.

'Vee-vee?' Gladys moved herself forward with her frame.

'Yes, Gladys. Are you alright?'

'Yes, but . . . I can smell something funny.'

'Oh? What kind of smell? Where's it coming from?'

'Down there, in the end room. You know, Doris's old room.'

'I'd better have a look. You stay here in the office, Gladys.'

Doris had died a few months earlier, and we were using her room as a temporary store-room until another resident moved in. I walked along the corridor. What if? It was not unknown for Catherine to sneak into Doris's room for a quick one in the warm.

Then, as I turned the corner, I saw smoke pouring under the door. I peered through the small window and could just make out a figure lying on the bed. I raced to the office phone, smashing an alarm button on the way. The admin block had to be notified first, then they contacted the emergency services. That was the procedure. I could hardly make myself understood on the phone, the alarm bell was so loud. The next half hour passed in a blur as I got the old ladies outside. Where were the other staff, for goodness' sake?

There wasn't time to ring another house for help. Those who could walk made their way outside, while I grabbed dining chairs and put them on the lawn in front of Birch House next door, our assembly point. The other residents were going to take longer to get out. One lady was so deaf she couldn't hear the alarm, but when she saw the smoke, she panicked, slid off the bed into her wheelchair and I was able to rush her out. I knew that there were six more ladies in the house. I grabbed more chairs, practically throwing them on the grass. Meanwhile the fire was taking hold and it was getting harder to see, despite the emergency lighting, and harder to breathe. I went as far round the house as I could, coughing, and managed to get four of the six out onto Birch lawn.

'Need a hand?' It was Jimmy from Birch. There was still no sign of Sandra or Nat.

'Please,' I gasped. Just then the fire exploded out of the lounge window, sending debris everywhere. The TV set must have gone. My ladies were by now far enough away – there was a garden between the houses – but they wailed in distress. Luckily it wasn't raining, but it was a chilly afternoon and nearly dark. Birch House staff were looking after the ladies, wrapping them in blankets, then taking them indoors.

Jimmy and I tried one last time to rescue Catherine and June, but it had now reached the stage where we couldn't go in again. At last a fire engine arrived, as flames engulfed the lounge area, crackling as high as the roof, and thick dark grey smoke poured from the main door. Jimmy and I stood in the road, exhausted, our hands on our knees.

'Who's inside?' shouted a fireman. A burnt joist crumpled into the building.

'Two women,' I shouted back. 'I think one of them started it by accident. I couldn't reach them.'

'Now you must stay here! We don't want any more casualties!'

They unravelled the hoses quickly and worked the water over the blaze. An ambulance pulled up, blue lights flashing. Then I caught sight of Sandra and Nat approaching. Nat was chewing as usual and their faces were yellow in the light from Alder House, now completely ablaze. The two women didn't show any sign of concern. Every minute or so, some part of the building would crash down, sending up sparks and groaning as if in pain.

'They're all out,' I said, still coughing. 'Except for June and Catherine. All the others are in Birch. Catherine was in Doris's room . . . I don't know if they'll make it.'

'You mean, they might be dead?' Sandra shouted over the noise.

'I don't know.'

'Weren't you keeping an eye on them?!' she thundered. A fireman looked round.

'I had been, then I had stuff to do in the office,' I said lamely. I was desperate to know where she and Nat had been for the last two hours, but I knew that if I vented my spleen it would be misinterpreted as illness and I would get that look which said "calm down!" along with an arching of the neck and a prolonged raising of eyebrows. This reaction could occur at any time actually, regardless of circumstances.

'Honestly, leave you alone for five minutes and this is what happens! If Catherine or June, or both of them die, it will go down on your report as negligence!'

A fireman appeared at the front door, pushing off his mask when he reached the road. Another followed him out. I wanted to ask if Catherine and June were OK, but thought better of it. An angry, greedy crackle filled the air and the orange light flickered over the buildings opposite. People were watching from the windows. Jimmy suggested we leave them to it now that Sandra was here and go and get a cup of tea.

A great cheer went up among the ladies when I entered the lounge in Birch, which was full to bursting, but Bill didn't acknowledge me. Jimmy and I sat in the office with our tea, trying to recover and get used to the idea that two residents might be dead. The other ladies from Alder would have to be split up. Sleeping arrangements would have to be made.

'What time does your shift end?' asked Jimmy.

'Oh, I forgot all about that! I was due off at four. What time is it now?

'Half past six. Want a lift home?'

'But what about June and Catherine?'

'There's nothing else you can do. You'll just have to leave it to the professionals.'

'I feel so guilty, Jimmy.'

'Hey, you did all you could. Nobody could have done more. If anyone should feel guilty, it's us in Birch for not coming out sooner. But we didn't know you were on your own.'

When we went back outside, the fire brigade had brought the blaze under control and Alder House was now a smoking black shell. The ambulance had gone. I went over to Nat, who was talking to one of the firemen.

'Where's Sandra?' I asked.

'Gone in the ambulance with Catherine.'

'Oh! So they got her out, then? What about June?'

Nat shrugged. 'Catherine's got bad burns. Might not make it either. You'd better watch out.'

After a couple of days off all round, Sandra, Nat, Liz and I were moved to work on Grove House. Sue and Sally went to Birch and Brian to Forest. The night staff were also divided up.

'Is Catherine going to be alright?' I asked Sandra.

'You'd better hope so,' she replied, leaning towards me, too close, confiding not a secret but a threat.

On my first day in Grove, I watched from the window as workmen erected a temporary fence round the Alder site. "Danger. Keep Out," read the signs. But the burnt shell could not be demolished until a thorough search had been made for June's remains. These were never found. I heard some time later that they were going to call a new house after her. A short service was held in the chapel and flowers appeared on the grass by the fence. About two weeks later, what was left of Alder House was razed to the ground.

Not only was Sandra desperate to find me lacking, she also wanted me to feel guilty. Since I knew that guilt feelings were part of my depression, I wanted to resist. Even if Catherine died, I was determined not to let Sandra open the white door again. She might not have been able to see it, but somehow she knew it was there, and kept scratching, working at it. If she succeeded in kicking it open, she would be able to declare a victory: "There you are! What did I tell you? She *is* useless!"

When I had first arrived at Alder House, bruised from my encounter with Bill (and another disciplinary hearing), I had made the mistake of repeating that I'd done nothing wrong. Now Sandra was seizing every opportunity to prove that I *had* done something wrong – several things, in fact.

With Catherine so ill, of course I was having doubts about my actions on the day of the fire. Perhaps I should have checked round one more time before I sat in the office. I fought these doubts by remembering that Sandra should have been on the house at the time, or at least told me where she was going. I couldn't make a formal complaint about Sandra's absence that day because I knew I would not be believed. I was low down in the Centre hierarchy and a nutter as well. Whichever way I looked at the situation, Sandra was in a stronger position.

She did have to work harder now, though, as she shared the role of Manager with Helen, who had done a stint on most of the houses but was at present managing Grove. I had begun to like Helen, especially when I found out her surname, and I looked forward to her shifts as a break from Sandra.

'Excuse me for asking, Helen,' I said, when we were alone in the office one day.

'But is your husband a psychiatrist?'

'He is indeed. Why?'

'Oh, I'd . . . heard of a Doctor Greenwood, that's all.'

'He sometimes gives talks for people like Mind. Perhaps that's how you heard his name.'

'Could be, yes.'

Helen smiled and went back to her paperwork. I liked her style. She must have known there was more to it, but her tact was a breath of fresh air.

When I'd had a morning shift with Sandra in charge, afternoon overtime on Forest put things back into perspective. Brendan knew what Sandra was like, and JD cheered me up in his innocent way. Ironically, I was given more responsibility when I came back to my original house than in my promoted state elsewhere. I wished I'd never left

Forest, because where I was now, it was assumed I was incompetent. Just as being trusted makes you confident, being regarded as a nobody makes you start to believe you are.

If ever I had a small success, it would be ignored or belittled by Sandra and her cronies. I would interrupt conversations about me when I went into the office, resulting in the muffled laughter typical of bullies. The fact that I had rescued the old ladies from the fire more or less single-handedly was never mentioned. What's more, I knew not to mention it, as I could predict the response: she would say that I was "just doing my job". Having to be so careful and guarded was a real strain. Sandra had me in a mental arm-lock.

Then one day, a month after the fire, Catherine was brought back to Grove House.

When he'd read this, Max wrote:

"Had she been in a position to influence those around her, many of the things that happened to Vee might have been avoided. For example, she would have known and been able to assert her rights against Sandra. But Sandra bullied her, wore her down over the months and destroyed her resistance, so that Vee just went along with whatever was happening, her feeling of powerlessness part of the nightmare she was living through. Vee was not in control of her situation, and she knew it. I am now, at last, beginning to see what I might be able to do for her."

18

Nancy

At the beginning of December, a new lady arrived to take up residence in Grove. Suitcases, boxes, a duvet and a teddy were carried in by members of her family. I looked out to see a large estate car, its hatch high in the air, and went to help.

'That's all now, thanks,' said one young man, out of breath. I didn't need to direct him along the corridor, as the shouts of, "Where d'you want this, Auntie?" and comments such as, "Phew, I could murder a cup of tea" left no doubt as to the location of Nancy's room.

I was told Catherine was still in a pretty bad way and needed a lot of care. If she had died, Sandra would have made sure I was out of a job, for certain. But even though Catherine had survived, there was no let-up in Sandra's daily campaign. She was pushing as hard as she could to provoke or break me. But the nastier she got, the more I resisted. Avoiding her as much as possible was the best method, so I spent longer with the residents. I wondered what more she could do.

I hadn't seen Catherine since her return, so I went along for a chat. She was lying on her bed, with dressings and bandages everywhere. Her face had patches of raw skin.

'How are you feeling, Catherine?'

'Oh, I'm alright Vee. Just me leg's a bit sore, see?' She lifted the corner of the dressing on her thigh.

I winced. 'That does look a bit sore, yes. What about the other burns?'

'Doc said I'll be scarred. It was a near go, dear. I 'haled a lot of smoke, too. Still coughing a bit, but . . . '

'It's amazing how you managed to escape in one piece, though! How *did* you do it?'

'Woke up; must've dozed off in there with a fag on – to find smoke, flames an' me cloves on fire. Rolled around a bit, like you see 'em on telly. Shouldn't've lay on that ol' bat's bed – p'raps that Doris wanted me to join her, silly old –' She tried to laugh, but ended up coughing. After the spluttering crescendo and climax, she groaned and patted her chest. 'Gi' me some oxygen, there's a dear.' She took a few breaths from the mask. 'So then I crawled out the room. Must've passed out. Next thing I knew I was in hospital an' it was *agony*, dear. Hope you never get burnt.' She lay back on the pillow and closed her eyes for a moment.

'Have you met the new lady, Nancy?'

'Can't really talk to 'er, can you? Seen 'er once, when she first got 'ere an' she wandered into my room.' She opened her eyes again. 'Course, at the moment I 'as to rely pretty much on what I 'ears, but I think she's a bit funny in the 'ead, if you ask me. That Sandra's done the right thing, lockin' 'er away when she's on duty.'

I smiled and let it go, but warning lights were flashing and I filed away the alarm I felt at this piece of information. 'Well, you had us all worried. And they cancelled the firework display this year. It didn't seem right somehow, what with poor June.'

Catherine went into another paroxysm.

'Anything I can get you, Cath?'

'Oooh, darlin', a cuppa would be lovely, but you'll 'ave to 'old it for me!'

A week later, Helen called a meeting at handover, when the residents had finished their lunch. Sandra sat in the corner of the office in her green coat, straight-faced and ready to leave. I had overheard an argument between the two managers the day before; it was always going to be likely with two women who were so different. I think it had something to do with Nancy, but I couldn't be sure. Sandra had shouted out something about her being "a nutter who deserves it", but then the door was slammed shut, so I didn't hear the rest properly. Today, we were all squeezed into the office, waiting for what Helen had to say.

'I have some important news for you. Some of you might already know that Bill, the manager of Birch House, passed away the night before last. Our thoughts are with Rosemary.'

'He woz sittin' at 'is desk, wozan 'e?' said Nat, fiddling with a thumb ring.

'I don't know the exact details,' Helen went on, turning towards Nat, 'but what I have to say is that Birch needs a new Manager for a short while. They have appointed me to stand in.'

I realised before she went any further that she might be taking some of us with her.

'So,' She looked round at the expectant faces. 'Nat: I think you need a change of scene, so you're coming with me.' Nat didn't seem impressed. 'Also Liz. Sue and Sally will be coming here from Birch. I think it's a good thing to have a shuffle round sometimes, yes? You get to know different managers' styles. I'll speak to the night staff this evening.' She smiled. I knew exactly what she was doing. I looked at my shoes, fighting off tears.

I watched our new resident over the next few days and I had to admit that Catherine was right about her: she was unwell. She would make strange comments at the table, swear and upset the others. Sometimes she burst out laughing for no apparent reason. Then one day she didn't come for meals.

'Where's Nancy?' I asked Sandra, who was back in total charge of a house again and loving every minute.

'In her room I expect.'

'But she hasn't been down for meals. D'you want me to check and see if she's OK?'

'Oh, stop worrying, will you! Everything's taken care of. And I don't want you going in her room. Do you understand? Earth to Vee! Leave her to me and to people who know what they're doing.'

From then on, Nancy remained in her room, the only one with the en suite bathroom, which Cath had wanted. I assumed food was being taken to her, but I was never allowed to participate in her care. None of the other staff would talk about her: there seemed to be a conspiracy. I wished I could get to the bottom of it, but once again, I knew nobody would believe me if I said anything outside the house, especially as Jack Marshall was so interested in Sandra.

It had now reached the stage where I was doing most of the work while Sandra and her new cronies sat talking and laughing. If I had to go into the office, they would stop as usual, and snigger. I would jump if Sandra called my name, fearing that I had made a mistake which she was going to point out with relish in front of the juniors. I must have deserved this but I couldn't work out why. It was a puzzle which made life even more difficult. At least the white door still seemed to be intact.

The only regular company I had were my flatmates and my neighbours, all of whom worked somewhere on the Centre of course – and Phisto. I didn't have the time, the energy or the transport to go much beyond Whyton on foot to get groceries, returning by taxi. Jim had bought me a bike to get around Squaremile; I didn't see myself ever owning a car again. Holidays were out too, apart from ones accompanying residents, which weren't really holidays at all. I simply didn't have the money: I was trying to pay off a large debt incurred as a result of going high.

It was impossible to find a fellow worker in whom I could confide safely. I had my diary, which was a good way to express emotions, but it couldn't answer back or question my perspective. I suppose I could have called Diane in Lexby, but I didn't want to bother her too often with a series of problems. Besides which she had a young son now and another baby on the way. I had been in touch with one of my own former teachers, Anne Sharp, recently, but getting to see her was difficult. However, I did still have Bella. While she was a nurse and not a friend, she had been visiting me for some time now and knew all about me. I let her in.

'Anyone else about today?'

'No, apart from the girl on nights,' I said in a stage whisper, closing the door which led to the bedrooms.

'How are things?'

I went to make some coffee. 'Oh, same as usual.' When I brought the cups in, I sat opposite Bella, who'd had her hair cut short. 'I like your hair!' I said.

'Thank you. Now bring me up to speed.'

'Well, Sandra hasn't changed. I still get the blame for everything. But the talk I was preparing to give when I last saw you went quite well. As you know, I was getting sick of negative attitudes towards people with mental health problems, so I asked Marge in the admin block, who's i/c staff training, if I could give this talk to staff about it. It's the teacher in me trying to get out.'

'Yes. Go on.'

I told Bella how Marge had let me use one of her rooms and how about fifty or so staff had turned up the previous Wednesday. I'd explained about neuroses and psychoses, bipolar and schizophrenia, etc., but I'd been particularly pleased with my idea for the beginning of the talk; having taught adults as well as children, I knew from experience that *involving* people got their attention. So first, I'd asked them to write down all the words and expressions they could think of which labelled someone who was ill. I got all the usual things: loony, nutcase, screw loose etc. Then I'd asked them to write down similar things which applied to someone with cancer. Surprise, surprise: there were none. Of course I'd then had to ask the big question: *why* is this the case?

'Sounds great! But were there any senior staff there, anyone who might be able to influence the mindset?'

'They were mostly juniors, I'm afraid. But I hope it still made them think.'

Bella then stated that she thought I confused Sandra. I didn't understand; she explained that Sandra didn't seem able to untangle the jealousy she must feel for my level of education from her view of my illness, which she clearly didn't understand. I recalled Bill's attitude. According to Bella, both of these things made her wary of me, which is partly why she was treating me so badly.

'I kind of half knew that.'

'Ah, these people!' Bella was fired up by the injustice she must have encountered every day. 'They think they're immune! Do they think you're *happy* being bipolar, and that you're ill just to annoy them?' She paused to sip her drink, then said: 'Vee, there's something I should tell you. There might come a time when I can't see you any more.'

I felt a sudden rush of anxiety. She went on: 'They're on the point of changing the system, to save money, of course. But the details haven't been thrashed out yet, so it could be a while. Don't panic just yet. I just thought I ought to warn you, that's all. Now,' She put down her mug. 'How do you feel about applying for a new job?'

'I have thought about it lately.'

'How about asking Sandra for a reference?'

I stopped myself from ridiculing this suggestion. 'Oh yes! I see! That way, if she wants to get rid of me, she'll be forced to say something positive!'

'Exactly. Give it a try. Ask her. You've got nothing to lose.'

I heard on the grapevine that Tim Clark, Health and Safety, was due to retire soon, and that Sandra had been tipped as his successor. I wondered if Sandra knew. It seemed likely. One cold morning when I had been sent to get the post, I caught sight of Tim Clark talking to someone I recognised, outside the admin block. It was Debbie from university. I had to say hello. Tim saw me coming and went indoors.

'Oh, hi Vee! It's been a long time!'

'Yes. About twenty years, I'd say!' We laughed. 'How long have you been working here? I haven't seen you around.'

'I've only been here a couple of months.' Debbie smiled. 'How are you?'

'Fine. You?'

'I'm OK now, but I've had ME, so I wasn't able to work for ages. But my dad knew someone who knew someone, as they say, and now I'm here.'

'Sorry to hear that. I mean, that you were ill.' I decided not to go into my history. 'Hey, d'you remember the Italian job? Four weeks round Italy with Theresa Jenkins!'

'That's right!' Debbie's eyes lit up. 'We were sick of her moaning about everything, weren't we? I'd just graduated, but you had to go back and be with her for another year! I do remember, yes.'

'Her bra and her chocolate got stolen in the Florence Youth Hostel!' I laughed again. But we were getting cold. 'Which house are you working on?'

'I don't work on the houses. I'm based here.' She pointed to the admin block behind us.

At that moment I realised she was smartly dressed, as I had been as a teacher. Care assistants, on the other hand, wore serviceable, casual clothes that were easily washed. The difference in our status was emphatic.

'Oh. Well if you ever want a chat, I'm in Grove House.' With that we parted.

She had a proper graduate role. And it became clear from her manner that Debbie would not want to meet me socially from now on. How was I ever going to climb back to where I thought I should be?

March came in like a lion, so Mum believed it would go out like a lamb. I approached the spring with my usual dread. Not that the white door opened every time, but this is when it was most likely. A different door, the one to Max's office, stood open instead. He smiled.

'Last time we met, you gave me a couple of your poems,' he began. 'I liked them. Can I keep them?'

'Yes. Remind me which ones they were.' We sat down.

'One about your brother and . . . one about a doctor.'

I felt strangely nervous, exposed. 'Oh, yes; keep them.' I had given birth to them and they had to make their own way in the world. But we were no more than doctor and patient now, weren't we? So I had the uncomfortable feeling that perhaps I shouldn't have let my guard down by showing him the poems.

He asked me how work was going of course. I said I tried really hard not to let it get me down, but I wished something good would happen for a change. Sandra, I said, found fault all the time, complete with long-suffering expression and upward-looking eyes. Max smiled. I said I could imagine her talking about me in meetings. I wasn't being paranoid; I knew they tried to undermine me whenever they could. While I might not have overheard anything, yet, I could feel a kind of poisonous vapour hanging in the air sometimes when I went in the office.

'Vee, er . . . they are concerned about your work.' Max coughed.

'What do you mean?' My heart thumped in horror.

'Well, they've sent me a list of questions about how your illness affects you. Don't be alarmed. I won't send any answers until you've seen them.'

I felt undermined. I wasn't sure how to react. I knew Max was on my side, but there was still something sinister in this.

He changed the subject. 'What about a new job, Vee? Perhaps it's time to move on.'

'I've already talked to Bella about that, and in fact I've got an interview next week.'

'Well done! What's it for?'

'A housemistress in a girls' boarding school.'

'Far from here?'

'Quite a way. The other side of London.'

'Well, I wish you luck. I suppose you might even get the chance to do some teaching again one day.'

'You never know. But Max –' I blurted it out before I was ready, '– I'm writing a book!'

'Wow! That's a major undertaking! When do you get time?'

'After shifts and on days off.'

'What's it about?'

'Oh, it's to do with someone who gets ill and loses her job
. . .'

'An autobiography?'

'Not quite, as I've made a lot of it up. Most of it, actually.
In fact it's . . . Max? Would you mind reading it? I mean,
when it's finished.'

'I'd love to.' He smiled and I saw again the clarity of his
eyes. For a second I was back at Diane's, at the party. He
picked up my notes from the desk next to him.

'Now . . . Vee.' He turned the pages and found what he
was looking for. He said my latest blood test showed my
lithium level was a *bit* higher than he'd like, so he wanted
me to reduce my dose by 200mg. Then I was to have another
test in a month's time; he would write out a blood sample
form out for me now. There was a pause while he hunted
one down.

'I met your wife.'

'Oh, did you? There you are. Are you happy with keeping
the rest of your meds the same?'

'Yes, especially at the moment.'

'Oh, spring, yes. Look Vee, we were . . . friends once. I
don't like to see you in trouble. Work is hard for you at the
moment and I want to stress that if there's any way I can help
– .'

'– I'll bear it in mind, Max. Thanks.'

A week later, he sent me the questions he'd mentioned
along with his answers, and I went through them with Bella.
As one might expect, it was evident that whoever had
compiled the questions had not the faintest idea about
mental illness, and certainly did not see me as a individual
with the same needs and hopes as anyone else. Equally
manifest in his responses was Max's professional approach,
which we both knew disguised his true feelings – about
Squaremile's practices I mean, of course.

The day after I saw Max, I was alone on duty with Sandra
and I would rather have been anywhere else on earth. After

the medication round, during which she treated me like a Starter Grade, I heard a heavy thump and a cry in the passage near the office. It was Florence, one of our larger ladies, who had fallen out of her wheelchair.

'I'll go and get the hoist, then, shall I?' I knew Grove shared one with Birch, and I had used one every day in Forest.

'No, don't bother. We can lift her.'

I couldn't believe my ears. On the Moving and Handling course I had attended, they said that to avoid the risk of back injury, lifting someone manually should only ever be attempted in an emergency, such as a fire. I knew all about that. And House Managers were supposed to set a good example, weren't they? Not for the first time, I was in a difficult position: if I fetched the hoist I would be going against Sandra's instructions, and if I helped her lift Florence, I would be going against good practice. I had to go against my better judgement in the end and we hauled the poor lady back into her chair in a most undignified way.

The important thing about this episode is that we were alone. This meant that Sandra could report that I couldn't be bothered to get the hoist because it was raining, or some other excuse. Alternatively, she could say that it had been *my* idea to lift the resident. I had no witness to the incident, nobody to back me up, so once again, I had to keep quiet. If nobody has any faith in you and your judgement isn't trusted, life is hardly worth living. The irony is that Squaremile wanted to be in the vanguard of good practice, with its recently granted "Investor in People" status. In that connection, I couldn't help thinking that once every organisation had achieved this award, it would become meaningless.

I travelled to the boarding school for my interview by bus and train, trying to clear my thoughts of the Sandra clutter. Whatever she decided to say or do was out of my hands. The world would keep on turning if I was sacked, wouldn't it? What could she do that was any worse than sacking me? At the same time, though, I knew that my confidence had suffered, and that was relevant right now.

March did go out like a lamb, as Mum had predicted. The sun was warm on my arm in the train. The interview went very well. It was refreshing to be back in a school environment: the old buildings, the spacious grounds and the trees, now coming into leaf, reminded me of Castlebrough. The Head of Boarding, Lesley Wallace, was a pleasant woman of about my age. To my surprise, she offered me the job then and there.

I was also invited to spend the following weekend at the school, to see how the house worked and meet the girls. I decided to wait until after that visit before I made any kind of announcement to my family, but I did tell Sandra that it was "likely" I'd got the job. Meanwhile, I was walking on air, feeling that Sandra could do no more harm. I felt protected by thoughts of a better future. For a while, in fact, she didn't have much to say to me at all; she probably didn't want to waste any more time on someone who was leaving.

But then my mood changed as it dawned on me that I had not mentioned a certain "little problem" at the interview. I knew I had to. So during the weekend visit, I asked for a private word with Lesley Wallace.

'The thing is . . . I get depressed sometimes.'

'I see,' she said, an almost imperceptible cloud passing over her face. 'I'll be in touch tomorrow. I've got your work number.'

I had seen that cloud before, at the infrequent interviews in those two years in West Pluting, and I remembered the trials of the kitchen table. I was pretty sure I knew what was coming. On Monday, the phone rang in Grove office.

'Hello, is that Miss Gates?'

'Speaking.'

'Oh, it's Lesley Wallace here.'

'Oh, yes.'

'I'm afraid I've got some bad news. We cannot offer you

the post of housemistress after all, in the light of what you told me.'

Although I had feared the worst, I still felt as if I'd been kicked in the head. I was trapped at Squaremile; my momentary elation had evaporated, my hopes of a triumphant escape were dashed. I felt as if I had swallowed a cold stone. Sandra asked me what was wrong; I told her.

'Pha! You must be used to bloody disappointments by now! And there'll be some more coming if I have anything to do with it!'

19

Trial

Max was feeling much stronger after two weeks' rest with Helen as his nurse. She, on the other hand, was looking very tired. She fell asleep as soon as her head touched the pillow these days, regardless of any noise from Jackson. Simon was keeping out of the way, burying himself in work or, at least Helen hoped, busy searching for alternative accommodation.

Meanwhile, Max had been allowed to go back to his once a week job at Squaremile. He could not help wondering if some of the problems the residents presented with had been caused by the conditions in which they lived. For the moment, he wanted to have a proper look at Vee's diary, rather than read on in the book; he hoped he might gain a more gritty image of the atmosphere at the Centre. The diary was still where he'd hidden it, behind the monitor. But first he felt like going for his favourite walk to clear his mind.

The cul-de-sac was a peaceful place: most of the children did their growing up at one private school or another. Today he was glad of his anniversary jacket. A robin landed on the gatepost at the back, its wistful song cutting through the cold air. As he approached, it bobbed, then flew away. The latch was almost frozen to the wood; he soon put his hands in his pockets, missing his gloves. The lane skirted two fields in a dip to his left. The animals he had seen here were now in their winter quarters. To the right was a row of hawthorns, the boundary of his neighbour's garden. A few lumps of old snow lingered in places. He breathed in the fresh air, not daring to think about the condition of his heart, but there was no pain. He got to the second field; behind both fields was woodland, which swept in a great arc round the far end and swallowed up the footpath. He walked about a mile, nearly to the edge of the wood, as far as the blackthorn bushes.

Back home he made a coffee (Helen had insisted they buy decaffeinated from now on) and headed up to the attic. He rubbed his hands and held the cup to warm them, then immersed himself in the diary. A short while later, he wrote:

"Evidence of Vee's fragility towards the end of her life could be found in her writing and was always linked with her treatment at work. She stopped work on her novel in June or July, but the diary went on until the beginning of September. Following her stay in Porteblanche from March to May of the previous year, she had been coping quite well for some time. As the months went by and the stress increased, however, she knew she would have to get out of Squaremile. I gave her a reference, but she experienced a series of rejections. Her diary goes into detail:

'This place is hell on earth. Nobody trusts me to do this bloody job which I could do standing on my head. They think I'm ill <u>all</u> the time! I don't stand a chance here. But nobody else wants to employ me either! God knows I've tried. I get all dressed up to go to some poky, tatty office in the back of beyond only to get the usual cloud pass over their faces and a rejection, either on the spot or through the post. [. . .] The latest thing on their minds, here, is whether I'm a danger to the residents!! You'd really think I'd invented mental illness. Sandra's got to be the worst manager on the planet. [. . .] I do the same work as everybody else. And how am I supposed to escape, if I can't get another job? What is there left for me?'

"Vee's frustration is clear. She had waited so long to get her promotion, only to end up with one bullying manager after another who saw her as nothing more than an unstable burden. I have the distinct impression that people wanted to see her become suddenly and violently unwell while on duty, justifying their concerns and meaning that what amounted to persecution could be overlooked in the way so typical of group cruelty.

"The pressures they exerted on Vee had but one goal: getting rid of her, by fair means or foul – not that fair means ever seemed to figure in the equation. Any legislation passed from now on to protect the employee against this type of treatment will come too late for Vee. The Union rep on site was blind to Vee's difficulties and it was plain that Squaremile did not know what to do with her. In the end, because the management could find no real fault with her work, they decided to engineer situations and *invent* faults."

Max had been given a good opportunity to step in and support Vee. When he'd seen her in March last year, her employer had just sent him the list of questions concerning her fitness for work. Suspicion, ignorance and fear on the part of Squaremile seems to have prompted this course of action: was Vee putting it on? Or if she *wasn't*, how were they supposed to cope? Just what was this "illness", anyway? (As if no information was available!) Max had sent Vee the questions, as promised, with his responses, before submitting them to the Personnel Officer.

Vee let him know that she was quite happy with what Max had written. Perhaps the most damaging aspect of all this, Max could see, was that Squaremile didn't seem to acknowledge that Vee had the same range of ordinary emotions as other people. The way the questions were worded was insulting. It made Max angry to think she could be dealt with and spoken about as if she were a dog, without human comprehension. And he regretted the likelihood that, since no amount of good work on Vee's part seemed to shift Squaremile's position, his responses would make any difference in this respect.

Since he no longer had a copy of the questions, shredded with a load of other papers recently, he wrote down what he remembered. They covered two sides of A4, with spaces for his answers, and they went something like this:

1. *Vee Gates has a diagnosis of manic depression. How does this affect her?*
2. *Does manic depression have an impact on Vee's work? If so, what?*
3. *Does manic depression make Vee a danger to herself or others, especially the residents in her care?*
4. *What are the effects of the medication Vee takes for manic depression?*
5. *Vee is taking increasing amounts of medication. What effect is this likely to have?*

The questions had angered him, not only because they showed total misunderstanding, but also because it was transparent that they were based on a set of assumptions, which took no account of Vee as an individual. No effort had been made, no research done into illness or drugs, presumably because they thought it was a waste of time. If the questions had been worded in this way, his replies would have been along these lines:

1. *Miss Gates has a diagnosis of manic depression, now known as bipolar disorder. She has spent time in hospital as a result, but was well on discharge. Bipolar disorder does not affect her otherwise.*
2. *Bipolar disorder has no adverse effects on Vee's work.*
3. *Vee is not dangerous. The residents are perfectly safe with her.*
4. *The effects of the medication for bipolar disorder are to allow the person to function normally and prolong the period between episodes of illness.*
5. *Vee is not taking increasing doses of any medication. She has remained on the same dose for several months. Her medication is reviewed on a regular basis and is carefully monitored.*

There was so much more he'd felt he wanted to say, especially in reply to questions 3 and 5. He realised that nobody at work had actually sat down with Vee and expressed to her face any concerns they might have. Perhaps they didn't think they would get a sensible answer. He'd found question 5 particularly offensive too on a personal level, implying as it did that he was not doing his job properly. None of Vee's drugs was addictive. He wondered what the "students" might have said on that subject.

The words of Vee's last two chapters, concerning Squaremile, spoke for themselves. Max remembered Vee as someone who knew the value of love, but who could never trust others to have the same feelings, which of course affected her relationships with men. She had written that she was *meant to be alone*. But he was not going to challenge Squaremile alone.

Now he read on in the book, as he suddenly remembered the importance of what was due to happen very soon.

I had just started my shift, the day after losing my chance to escape to a boarding school from Squaremile. Sandra stood in the doorway of the office in Grove. She wanted me to come to a meeting with her. I was puzzled. She told me I would find out what it was about when I got there. She ignored all my questions from then on, and I followed her down the corridor to what was known as the teaching room, speaking less and less as I realised it was pointless, growing silent and anxious, like an animal being led somewhere. A dog on a lead . . .

The first person I saw was Mr Montgomery, the Chief Executive. He stood to greet Sandra with raised eyebrows and a nod, then sniffed as he sat back down and adjusted his reading glasses, papers in hand. Jack Marshall and Tim Clark were there, on either side of the CEO. They wore dark suits and were also studying their mysterious, rustling sheets of paper. It was as if I didn't exist until I had taken my seat in front of them. Sandra thrust a copy of what they were looking at into my hands, tutting as if I had forgotten one given previously, then sat by the door.

It suddenly became clear to me why I had not been challenged quite as much as usual over the last few weeks on Grove. It had nothing to do with my job prospects or with any kind of relaxation of "prison rules". The fact was, they had been watching me and making notes. My heart sank.

'This meeting has been called,' Jack Marshall announced, 'to examine certain irregularities in your work, Miss Gates, over the past few months. Please read the first item on the list.'

Jack Marshall put on his reading glasses. His Birmingham accent rang in my ears and I could hear my pulse alongside it. My blood pressure made me a bit deaf. I began to tremble.

'According to this item, you have been making dangerous errors in the administration of medication. Have you anything to say?'

For a second it felt as though everyone in the room was far away, like a remembered nightmare. But then someone moved impatiently and I knew I had to say something. But what? I was condemned before I'd entered the room.

'That's not true,' I managed, trying to control my trembling.

Jack went on: 'If it's not true, why has it been brought to our attention? Are you saying that your boss has made up these . . . difficulties you're having?'

I couldn't answer. One by one the other items on the list were read out and I made a feeble attempt at defending myself. Had I been given the sheet beforehand and time to prepare, I might have done a better job. But then, they knew that.

'Number eight on the list.' With every new allegation, Jack was distancing himself from me like a prison officer from those he regards as worthless. 'This concerns the fire at Alder House. You were responsible that day. Sandra had trusted you by leaving you in charge, and yet through your negligence, one resident died and another was seriously injured. What have you got to say about that?'

'I . . . did what I could.' It was pointless. Everything was rigged in Sandra's favour.

There was a long silence, during which glances were exchanged that weren't hard to read.

'The last item relates to an incident on Grove where you refused to fetch a hoist from Birch House next door, in order to help lift a lady who had fallen over. Now, you attended the course on Moving and Handling, didn't you?'

'Yes.'

'So you are aware of the importance of using the correct equipment?'

'Yes.'

'So why did you insist that the lady could be lifted manually? Sandra had to go and fetch the hoist herself!'

'It's not true!'

Jack Marshall was standing up now, agitated.

'According to you, none of this is true! Who are we to believe? A trusted House Manager with years of experience or you, with your mental health problems?'

I knew there would be a reference to that at some point. Again, I could not answer. I hoped my memory lapses were not responsible if I *had* been making mistakes. It was spring . . .

Sandra spoke for the first time: 'This list was compiled from reports by staff on Alder and Grove, and my own experience of Miss Gates's behaviour at work. I am, however, willing to give Vee one more chance. Do you agree?'

Mr Montgomery and the senior managers looked at each other and held a brief, whispered conversation. I knew precisely what Sandra was doing. She was on the verge of victory, of getting what she'd been working towards for months. I wondered how long ago the managers had been given the document. She had no doubt pretended to be at her wits' end because of me. Now, in these moments, her apparent magnanimity would shift the responsibility for this meeting and its consequences neatly on to the three men, while creating a firm belief in her decency and humanity.

'I try to help my staff as much as possible.' Sandra was gloating almost uncontrollably, trying oh so carefully to channel the fire of anticipation into making absolutely certain that the roots of this belief she was planting were sound; her voice was soft and her tone obsequious. 'And Vee has had a lot to cope with, poor thing. There must be more we can do.'

Tim Clark stood up. 'We are satisfied that you have done everything in your power to help Miss Gates. Unfortunately, given what we have heard today, we believe it is in everyone's interest to terminate Miss Gates's employment with immediate effect. The warnings she has received over the years have obviously done nothing to improve her performance and so we have reached the end of the line.'

'Oh, Vee! I'm so sorry!' Sandra sighed. Then she smiled at me. It was an empty, cold smile; in her eyes was no care or concern, only cold triumph and contempt. She had won.

Max recalled how distressed Vee was when she saw him for an extra appointment at the beginning of July.

'How are you?' This was his professional question to see if his own perception matched that of the patient.

'Oh, Max.' She clasped her hands in her lap. 'I don't know what I'm going to do.'

'Why? What's happened?'

'They've kicked me out. But it's not as simple as that. We had this meeting.'

'Bella mentioned that. Go on.'

'I didn't know it was going to happen and I didn't know what it was about until I got in the room and saw that piece of paper. Sandra wouldn't tell me.'

Vee described the meeting, showing how it was a "put-up job". The words she used to describe her boss were not in the least complimentary. He was glad he had not contributed any fuel to this fire; he had made sure the answers to those questions had been positive. If they thought he was protecting his patient, so be it.

'Vee, I'm sorry to hear about this. But surely it's illegal to subject someone to such an ordeal. Is there no way you can claim unfair – or constructive – dismissal?'

She explained that she'd signed an agreement; they'd paid her to keep quiet. They'd actually said that's what the money was for. He was shocked and pointed out that this was an admission of guilt. She should take some kind of action against them. Vee was silent for a moment. Then she said she couldn't do it. She wasn't strong enough. It was too much for her.

'That's what they want! They're counting on that.'

But Vee was defeated. 'I was suffocated in that room by their combined will. Who's going to believe me? Oh, it must be my fault. Nobody else seems to find life so difficult to deal with!'

Max knew that Helen would have played no part in this outrageous episode. She probably didn't even know what was going on, so tied up was she with reorganising Birch. He couldn't interfere either.

Max found out that Vee was allowed to stay in her tied accommodation until 31st July, so that when they'd met at the start of the month, she was waiting to hear where and when she would be rehoused, thanks to Bella's foresight. Vee had expressed anger, grief and anxiety while in Max's office, but these emotions were entirely appropriate; he had seen nothing more sinister on the horizon. Bella saw her twice before she moved, as Max had advised her of the extra support she would need. On 1st August, Bella told him, Vee moved into a flat in Cressington, a district of Howcester at the opposite end of the town from the hospital. Max read more entries in the diary:

'This flat is a quarter of what looks like a 60s semi, on the ground floor, so no stairs for Phisto to worry about. Seems like a quiet area, good for writing. Ron, Jim & friends helped move. Place completely bare: no carpets, curtains, cooker or fridge. Can use some of pay-off money, but Mum said she'd buy carpets & wardrobe. Bella will help with getting benefits, but warns they're not instant, so will

have to live off rest of Sq [sic] *money. Have gone down in the world, not up! But will start again looking for job.'*

In spite of everything, Vee seemed optimistic at this stage. Perhaps it was a kind of rebound from the pressure she'd been under. Or it could have been her innate courage, her need to keep going. Max wrote:-

"It appears that there are businesses where those in charge seem to have convinced themselves that company policy meets all the conceivable needs of their present and future employees (a situation reminiscent of Orwell's *1984*), so that this policy is implemented automatically, without further thought, yet with a silent, perhaps even unconscious gratitude on the part of the management at being allowed to discriminate behind the scenes, possibly with such frequency that their actions become regarded as normal, acceptable, in any event certainly unquestioned.

"In such an environment, people like Vee are doomed to failure. The seeds of prejudice can flourish behind closed doors when job applicants are required by law to declare their disabilities. Such legislation merely fortifies business policy which excludes people. And in the end, neither proof of discrimination nor weapon against it are readily available to those interviewed, or indeed those already employed. More silent victories pass unnoticed.

"Vee was not only disappointed in the workplace. She realised too that, as in the case of her brother, people she knew well couldn't understand why ultimately she was not working. This often happens; relatives and close friends cannot believe that someone they know and love can be so very ill, or so very stigmatised. Then, of course, what they say and do is unhelpful to the patient."

Max returned to the diary.

'It's no good. Whatever I try for, even stacking shelves, I cannot break through into work. I'm going to have to find other ways of occupying my time.[. . .] Why should I, for the sake of appearing to be brave, keep subjecting myself to a series of rejections? Life should hold more than this. It's no fun. If you go part-time, you lose out too.

'I keep going back to the things that led up to that meeting. Stupid, I know, but I was chatting to Nat [. . .] in the office and trying to describe what it felt like to want to kill yourself & how I could just take all the drugs in the medication trolley. Of course I wasn't serious – why would I do that with loads of people about? But Nat hid her anxiety. Then, as I found out later, she rang for Jack Marshall to come to the house. I remember him dropping in, but thought nothing of it at the time; it was not that unusual, especially when Sandra was on. This was during the lead-up period, the quiet weeks when (as I now know) the staff were busy making notes about me for her ladyship.

'Squaremile employed me knowing about my illness. That didn't stop the disciplinary hearings, warnings – and then the meeting. Too much significance was attached to my every word and action in the lead-up. [. . .] Job hunting is now a nightmare. And as for the courses designed to help you back to work, why do they always assume that if you're unemployed you are illiterate, uneducated and unskilled? Someone like me is assumed to be stupid or dangerous – or both. What I need is a fair employer [. . .]

'I know Jim means well. He's always been anxious to help when I'm ill, but then he expects me to carry on afterwards as if nothing's happened! We can never discuss it properly. There's always this charged atmosphere, as if he thinks I'm a fraud because I've stopped trying for jobs. Bella knows how difficult it is. Of course I would work if I could, but there comes a time when you've tried everything in your power and you have to say, Enough is enough. At least nowadays I'm not being judged and monitored all the time.'

Keeping a diary was obviously cathartic for Vee. Max remembered when he first met her, at Jeff's party in Lexby. She was an attractive, ambitious career woman. They had watched the sunset together, drinking champagne. They thought their separate futures were decided and secure, at the same time wishing the future could have been shared.

20

New Home

From my front door here in Cressington I can watch people walking their dogs in the field which slopes upwards from our lawn. Bella had been right to make sure I was on the Housing Association's waiting list for a flat; she must have known others who had been stranded by employment disasters. These used to be council houses, built in a hurry in 1960. They look like semis, but they're actually blocks of four flats. At the back, a row of tall hornbeams separates the garden from a building site. They remind me of the dignified trees outside Tor ward. I sometimes think about that place and wonder if the ghosts of long-dead inmates haunt the new occupants of the luxury flats.

I like it here because I don't have to share, except with Phisto. I like it here because the danger of spring is over. I like it here because I don't need to think about Squaremile all the time. They tried to kick open the white door. Just because they've stopped kicking doesn't mean there's no pain, but at least they're not here to see it or to judge me. They are miles away. Mum and Bella have seen it. And Squaremile's money doesn't stop me remembering: forgetting what happened is impossible.

I know that everyone, every person who ends up in this street, has had some kind of major upheaval in their life. I have not spoken to many neighbours yet though, because there is scarcely room in me for anyone else at the moment. Even when Jim arrives, with Matthew – who's grown a lot – with a bunch of flowers, the edges of me bristle with anxiety, which can feel more like terror. There is just enough room to skim the top of his news. He does not really see into me because I keep the outside clear of signs, things which might make him ask difficult questions.

We wander about in the garden for a few minutes. It is sad that Matthew is growing up without a mother, but Jim seems calmer these days. Sophie's death is quite a long time ago now, and Matthew is at secondary school. Jim has aged; he probably thinks the same of me, but each of us knows why.

Still, Jim has not lost interest in women; he comments on the figure of the eighteen-year-old neighbour who is sunbathing. When we've gone indoors, I tell him I think she's called Danielle. Jim raises his voice above the noise of the kettle.

'It's not a bad place, really, is it? From what I've seen on my travels, you could have done a lot worse.'

His *travels*, in his line of work, must have included some pretty rough areas. But every time I have a visitor, I see the flat as if through their eyes, as a disappointing place to end up. Yes, I was washed up here, or rather thrown here after the blast: I didn't choose this flat. They just said, "here's your flat" and left. I supposed I would just have to get used to it, because there was nothing else. I had lost the right to choose . . . And I would have to go without, and I would have to decorate it, and I would have to . . .

'Jim, I'm not feeling too good. Sorry. Think I need a sleep.'

'Well, we'll go and see Granny and Ron, shall we Matthew? But we can't stay too long . . . '

Nobody has been aware of the weather until there is a loud clap of thunder: Matthew runs to the window to spot the next lightning strike. As the rain begins to fall more fiercely, there is a shriek from outside and Danielle knocks on the door. I have to let her in, but I am stretched to my limit of being with other people. I cannot prolong my endurance much more.

'Oh, sorry! Didn't fink it was goin' to rain that quick! Couldn't get home in time!'

'Come in.'

She clutches her towel, covered in bits of grass, as

someone turns up the rain volume even higher and a flash fills the living room with light. Dogs are barking, people running. Nobody realises I am beginning to drown. I take a breath and introduce Jim. Matthew tries to smile at Danielle, but then jumps as another thunderclap rumbles about overhead. Danielle, sitting on the sofa, is a little uneasy in her bikini and spreads her towel over her knees.

'I'll go when it eases off a bit,' she says, then her mobile rings, a pop song I've never heard. 'Yep. I know! Bit sudden, wasn't it!' She slips off her sandals, makes herself at home. Phisto goes over to her and sniffs her outstretched hand as she talks on the phone. The thunder doesn't bother him as much as it used to, now he is a bit deaf. He used to hide under the bed . . . 'I'll see ya later then. Bye!' Danielle shuts her phone with a click and there is another bright flash. The lamp flickers. Jim counts aloud to Matthew: the storm is three miles away. The rain hammers on the window and my own storm still rages. It needs all my strength not to show it. Now Danielle pulls the towel round her shoulders and looks at me.

'So, what do you do with yourself all day, Vee? I mean, you don't go out to work, do you?' They had been watching. I thought so.

'Oh, I keep myself busy. I'm writing a book at the moment. What about you? What do you do?'

'I'm a care assistant, down the road at the old people's home. But why haven't you got a job then? Her pale eyes, smooth skin and long fair hair are the picture of innocent youth, though I suspect she is far from innocent. If I didn't colour my hair nowadays I would be white, like Ron.

'I mean, you're an intelligent woman,' Danielle goes on, drilling my head, 'I'd have thought it'd be easy for you to get a job.'

'It's a long story, but I've been ill,' is the only scrap I can throw her.

Danielle turns. 'Jim, isn't it?'

He nods.

'D'you mind me askin' what you do for a living?'

I could tell this was all being filed away for the benefit of others.

'It's kind of similar to what you do.' He smiles politely, closing ranks with me.

'Oh.' Danielle lacks the maturity to pursue either of these two mysteries, and we know that she doesn't want to appear too nosy. Nor is she keen to stay any longer than necessary.

A short while later she jumps up. 'Look, it's practically stopped raining. I'd better be going. Said I'd meet my boyfriend. Better get changed too!' She giggles. 'Can't go into town like this, can I? The mad bikini woman from Cressington. Still, we're not that far from the nut-house, are we?' She laughs, pushes her feet into her sandals and pulls the towel off her shoulders, leaving grass on the sofa which she doesn't seem to notice. 'Nice talking to you.'

I collect the cups and put Jim's flowers in water. Matthew finishes the drink I gave him. I haven't felt strong enough to have a proper conversation with him today, but there'll be other times.

'She could've made it to her own flat,' I say. 'I think she wanted an excuse to find out about me, so she could report back.'

'Quite likely,' Jim replies. 'But don't take her too seriously, Vee. She's very young.'

'Oh, she doesn't bother me.' I try to pick up some of the grass, then sit in one of the second-hand chairs. Its rounded wooden arm-rest bears the scars of its previous life: two heat rings from ancient cups of tea at an unknown address.

'Are you OK, Vee? You seem . . . tense.'

'I am. Look, I'm not being horrible, but I really need a bit of time on my own. Take Matthew to Mum's and say I'll ring her in the morning. Sorry, Jim.'

He gives me a significant look. 'OK.'

'Oh, before you go – here. I ran off a draft of the book for you to read. Would you like it?'

'Thanks, Vee. Should be interesting.'

I kiss Jim, but Matthew doesn't want my kiss. My baby – Max's baby, would have grown up by now. I had to stop myself wondering about what might have been. I don't intend to be around when Max reads about it.

I slept. It must have been about seven o'clock that evening when the phone woke me. It was just one of those annoying cold calls, so I hung up. The tension in me seemed to have unravelled itself, but the background feeling was still there. I tried to analyse it. I suppose I had trained myself to do that since the psychology sessions with Lucy. There was grief and helplessness. There was fear. There were the taints of everything that had happened which should have been different, better, marking me like the scars of a whip.

I expect Mum will pop in again tomorrow, now I'm only ten minutes' drive away. She loves to help me make this my home, because she senses I don't care about it yet. We go shopping, we go out for lunch – something we never used to do when I was younger, until the time she stayed with me in West Pluting. She wants to help in practical ways. She says Ron will help me decorate, but in the end I have to say I'm not ready. Why? She asks. It's a difficult question to answer without dragging the past back on to the scene and risking tears.

Perhaps I will be ready in a few months.

21

Helen

Simon's son Jackson had been stealing money from Helen's purse, to buy alcohol. When she found out, she had a row with him and his father while Max was in hospital; she'd kept this from him so as not to worry him when he was ill. But they were both glad when Simon announced that he'd found somewhere else to live. He wouldn't say where, but he was very apologetic and assured them he would repay the money as soon as he could.

Max knew Simon was finding things difficult; he hadn't even charged him any rent. But he couldn't help feeling disappointed and taken advantage of. Max tried to find Simon, who had not been in to work as expected for several days. However, despite his efforts to track him down, Max never saw or heard again from his former colleague, or Jackson. In fact they were on file as missing.

Helen was sitting in the reclining armchair the next morning, looking pale.

'Are you alright, darling?'

'I've got a terrible headache,' she said in a hoarse voice of suffering. He offered to get her some painkillers, but she said she'd just taken some. 'Besides which, we're nearly out.'

'You've got to be OK for tonight, my love.'

'What's tonight? Oh, yes. Your farewell dinner at Lisette's. I'll try. Max? Could you pop to the chemist's for me?' She closed her eyes and he didn't feel he could broach the subject of Vee's book. They only had one more chapter to read. He wanted to know more about what happened with Sandra; in particular, he wanted Vee's description of how things were between Sandra and Helen, followed by what Helen herself felt, of course.

He felt that writing about Vee had eased his guilt. It was probably just the act of expressing himself on paper that created this illusion. This led to the recognition that he hadn't really started work. It would have been too easy, in his profession, to become inured to individual suffering, to diagnose, treat and send people on their way without feeling their pain. Of course a degree of detachment is necessary. But in focusing on Vee, he had rediscovered why he became a doctor in the first place.

He didn't know if Simon had ever had that experience. An unexpected sense of relief, at the departure of their guests, was overshadowed by a new concern however: Helen's health. But they were both tired; he hoped that with quiet nights and good rest, she would soon be back to her old self. He began to wonder if he hadn't taken her for granted, for years.

Lisette's, where they had had their anniversary meal, was his favourite restaurant. Set back from the road and about twenty minutes away by car, it had a well-known chef, so whatever you chose was sure to be top quality, both visually and on the palate. Sue, a fellow consultant, and her husband Chris, a clinical psychologist, both from Porteblanche, picked them up at seven. The car was filled with perfume, smart jackets and sparkles on the ladies. Helen always felt a little left out on such occasions, and today she had to make a special effort for Max as well. Aware of this, Max told her how lovely she looked and didn't make any demands while they talked shop, the easiest option nevertheless.

'So, Max: how's retirement?' Chris turned slightly in the passenger seat and smiled.

'D'you want the psychological version?'

Chris laughed. 'Any version you like.'

'Well – Helen will back me on this – I've been a bit lazy so far.' he glanced in her direction and saw her raise her eyebrows briefly, then turn away. From the driving seat Sue chipped in.

'I think you probably deserve a rest. This job can really take it out of you. Helen told me you had a heart attack. Are you OK now?'

'Fine.' Max noticed that Helen was still staring out of the window into the night, so he squeezed her hand. They pulled up in the restaurant car park. When they had ordered, Sue said she had some news.

'Did you know, Max, that the Porteblanche wing is set to close in six months' time?'

'No, I didn't. Where will everybody go?'

'It was announced last week and should be in the local rag by now. They'll have to go to Okebury, which is where I'm off to, or Marmston.'

'But Marmston's *miles* away, the other end of the county!' Max could foresee all kinds of problems. 'I don't suppose there'll be any more beds available either. When will they realise that closing a place down doesn't take away the need for it!' Helen rubbed his knee under the tablecloth. 'Do they imagine that if they go round closing hospitals – and it's not just psych wards – there won't be any more sick people? Where will it end? Hospitals seem to be going the way of post offices!'

The news about Porteblanche put Max in a bad mood and he did not enjoy the evening as much as he might have done after that. From Sue's expression, she realised she'd made a faux pas; it was Max's special evening, after all. Meanwhile he recalled something Vee had written: she thought that every time she grew attached to a place, or it had some significance for her, someone would come along and tear it down. He knew what she meant. The worst part though is not just being powerless, but being powerless when those who *do* have the power don't know what they're doing.

Helen's behaviour concerned him too; she had slipped out to the ladies to take some more tablets and she had nearly fallen over when she stood up from the table. She hadn't drunk anything. Sue and Chris came back home with them after the meal and didn't leave until about midnight, by which time it was too late to embark on any major discussion. Helen was distant, disconnected from him, but at least he thought he knew why.

Tuesday morning came round again, and his weekly session at Squaremile. He did not see Helen at work. As usual, he borrowed one of the offices in the Day Hospital, and care assistants brought residents over for their appointments. He was glad there were no new cases today; the work was straightforward, checking how people were doing on their medication etc. In the evening Helen seemed a bit better; she was tidying the bedroom.

'Darling . . . Tell me about Sandra Wheatley.' He sat on the bed.

'Why do you want to talk about her?'

'Because I think that if prejudice can only be tackled on an individual level, she's got to be that individual.'

'Shall I tell you something you really don't want to hear?' She sat next to him.

'Since you put it like that, how can I refuse?'

'Sandra's got her promotion. She's now Health and Safety Officer, in place of Tim Clark. Everyone's wondering whose bed – .'

'– D'you really think she'd do that? It's bad enough hearing she's been promoted. SHIT!' He thumped the mattress.

Helen went on, 'When we worked together, that is, on opposite shifts, on Grove for a little while before I went to Birch, it didn't take me long to work out that she'd cut corners wherever she could and that she had favourites on the staff. She could take an instant dislike to people and once you were in her bad books, that was it.' Helen sighed. 'You know, I should really have reported her when I was there then. I was sure she wasn't doing her job properly. But getting evidence is always the tricky part.' Helen stood up, wanting to finish tidying while she felt able to.

'D'you think anyone will ever see through her?' Max asked.

'Well, I think that's where you and I come in.' Helen began plumping up the pillows. 'I'm thinking back over several House Managers' meetings. She doesn't contribute a thing in the way of new ideas, just finds fault with what other people say. Then she pretends it doesn't matter to her what's decided. It wouldn't be so bad if she could come up with something herself to . . . ' Helen shrugged, ' . . . solve a problem, or . . . but she's so negative, she puts a damper on the whole meeting. Frankly, people are quite glad if she can't come. And another thing: I was over in Grove one lunchtime and saw her picking up a sausage from the floor and putting it back on a resident's plate.'

'Hmm. Shows how much respect she has for them.'

'It's what we *don't* see we should worry about. Oh, and she still gets her month off!'

His writing desk was piled high with papers and folders, some of which belonged to Grace. Unfortunately, the back numbers of *Shrink* had not obeyed their own imperative either, but he hated throwing them out. He moved the old patterned rug which they'd given up on downstairs because it always "walked" to where it was most inconvenient. Then he sat in the creaky chair at the other desk where the computer waited and switched on the lamp. He found Vee's diary again, tucked behind the monitor, and opened it near the end.

'I can feel it starting again. A shadow that is inside me, not outside. It tightens my fists and I see two long thin tubes from them to the world, with papery leaves fluttering at intervals. They are very sensitive to what's going on. If anything disturbs the calm here they become agitated and start to entwine. They must not do that. Then I realise they are the ivy pulling me towards the white door. I don't want the anger it brings. I must stay indoors because everyone looks at me when I go out. I am ugly and I hate myself. I ought to know better. They're laughing at me now . . . '

There were only two more entries after this, but they were barely legible. This showed Vee descending into psychosis. She must have experienced fluctuations in mood and aware-ness, because when they met in August – for the last time –

he had not detected any psychosis. Anxiety was the predominant symptom then. Her mission was to deliver her manuscript. Naturally, he was concerned about her, but he could not have predicted what was to follow a month later.

Bella had, however, warned him that things were not going too well, so perhaps they should have had Vee back in. It's never easy, and as Simon had once pointed out, psychiatry is an inexact science, but these are human lives. He recalled what Bella said:-

"She's definitely having a depressive mood swing. Trouble is, she never realises how bad it's getting until it's too late and there's only one option left."

He asked if she thought Vee should come in, and Bella sighed. She said she was seeing her more often at the moment – the next day in fact – so she would keep him up to date. Three weeks later, Vee was dead. Filled once again with remorse at his delay, Max began reading the last chapter of *Doors Closing*.

22

Anne

Mum came over the next day, and I appreciated her continuing efforts to brighten up my flat. The trouble is, I can't seem to shake off the echoes of Squaremile, of black thoughts and bad experience. I went on writing about feelings like this in my diary.

Towards the end of my time at Squaremile, I got in touch with one of my former teachers, Mrs Sharp, who still lives in Howcester. Anne was very kind, and didn't judge me. Very soon she allowed me to put aside the outdated teacher-student relationship and we got together now and then for meals or walks. She visited me the last time I was in hospital. Today I wanted to put forward some ideas, think aloud with her before I finalised certain things in *Doors Closing*.

Anne is not very tall and has short, iron-grey hair. She welcomed me into her home made large by those absent. She is a widow, whose son and daughter are both married with families. In all the rooms downstairs, up the staircase, along the landing, in every bedroom, even in the cloakroom are books, so that each sound is muffled into a solidity of learning, a quiet dignity normally exclusive to second-hand bookshops. I am reminded also of my feelings when in France, the almost tangible breadth of the country, the heavy vastness. There is something about collections of books though that always makes me *feel* the august presence of knowledge, like a visit to an Oxford college. At Anne's house there is also a huge leafy plant in each main room. We sat in the living room with our coffee.

'I want to write something about how things have changed,' I began. 'I don't mean the obvious lack of a job. I mean, well, changes in my life brought about by how other people see me.'

'Does it matter to you what other people think?'

I needed to convey the importance and permanence of the changes. Anne was doing her best to understand, but her reply did rather suggest that for a moment, she saw me as a teenager in crisis. On the other hand, I could regard it as a simple acceptance of my situation, so I could not afford to sound hostile. I explained what I meant: until I got ill, people had taken my abilities for granted. So had I. Now, it seemed that having a breakdown meant I was weak through and through in their eyes. It is regarded as a terrible flaw in your very soul; even your moral standing is called into question. I hadn't understood this to start with, because I couldn't see anything wrong with my mind when I was well. Anne remembered how I'd been top of my year at 'A' Level, and could see that nobody would expect anything less.

'It must be difficult,' she said. 'I can see that things are very different now.'

'Yes, but it's not just that. It's to do with work, and people's attitudes. When I noticed the difference in the way people saw me, I was surprised at first, because in my head, nothing had changed. To me, I was the same person I'd always been – putting aside changes in my attitude, of course. Then I became frustrated at being treated differently. Now I'm resigned to a future without a job because other people have all the power.'

Anne came over and opened a window near me. It was a hot day and she didn't have a fan. 'I'm listening,' she said.

'That's a summary. Apart from my family, whose increased worry is the only change, I think I can identify two distinct attitudes towards me. I have to add that it's not really *me* any more that people are seeing, but a kind of walking illness with my face on it.'

'That's good!' Anne laughed.

I attempted to describe the two attitudes. The first type made no allowances whatsoever. People would turn their backs on me, scorning my weakness. They were the "pull yourself together" brigade. I felt the weight of their censure. With the second attitude, I went on, people expected *too little* of me, all the time, were too indulgent, even when I was well between episodes. In the past, when it was taken for granted that I was "normal", expectations of me had always been high, and I usually delivered. But now the jury was out, I said. Anybody could be in either of these two camps: old friends, new friends, nurses – and even doctors.

'I'd never really thought of it in that way,' said Anne, who had been clutching her coffee mug while she listened. 'Then again, I have been lucky enough not to have to formulate my relationships quite so clearly. So, which group do I belong to?'

'Oh, Anne! I count you as part of my family!'

She smiled. 'Thank you. But Vee, there is something I know for certain: you have a mother who hasn't given up on you, and a good step-dad and brother.'

She was right, of course. I mustn't forget that I was lucky in that way. I'd also had a good CPN who'd made sure I got somewhere to live and sorted out my benefits. My family had made sure I'd got off to a good start in the new flat. But with these physical needs met, I had to think about where my life was going.

'More coffee?'

'Not just now, thanks.'

'Let's go back to the Two Attitudes you were on about. Can you give me some examples. Only, I can't undo your summaries without a bit of help.'

'Well, the "pull yourself together" brigade, the PYTB, are usually, but not always, people you don't know very well. They are dismissive; they might be employers. The soft ones, the people who expect too little, the wet "I understand" group, are generally viewing your future with so little hope that you become insignificant – just another sick person whose opinions can be ignored.'

'Forgive me for saying this, Vee, but these two attitudes sound like two sides of the same coin. If you're not expected to be able to do anything, then surely you're being dismissed, or have I overlooked something?'

I thought for a moment. 'You see! This is why I needed to talk to someone with an unbiased brain! I think you're right.'

Anne smiled.

'But I went to see Mrs Finn too, around the time I got in touch with you. I was trying to gather allies.'

'Oh, yes, she taught English.'

'I told her all about being bipolar and the problems at work. I had not been ill for a while. D'you know what she said?'

'Go on.'

I tried to copy Leila Finn's note of weary cynicism: '"Oh, Vee! Don't you think it's high time you put all this behind you, for God's sake!" That wasn't all, but by the end of the conversation, I knew that Mrs Finn would never understand. She seemed to regard my eight bouts of illness as nothing more than an adolescent phase.'

'But it *is* difficult to understand, Vee, if you've never had any problems of your own, or known somebody.'

'Fine, true, but that's surely a first class reason *not* to be dismissive! I've never had appendicitis, but I still acknowledge that it occurs and that it's painful!'

Anne laughed.

'There's one other important thing about the PYTB, which concerns work. They despise me for not having a job. I'm just lazy. But would *they* employ me? They see it as my fault I'm out of work, but they've got me labelled up.'

'That's hypocrisy.' Anne stood up and took our mugs from the low table. 'Would you like to stay for lunch?'

'That would be nice. Thanks, Anne. Sorry to bang on, but – .'

'– It's fine, it's fine. Don't worry! You obviously needed it! Come out and sit in the kitchen while I make a start.'

I followed her along the hallway, its pale green walls lit from behind us by the glass front door and then after a dark corner, by the huge kitchen window, adorned with a row of

herbs on the sill including basil and thyme. I noticed a tray
of seedlings whose tiny pairs of leaves resembled tilted
green chairs. Rows of small but mature trees, some with
apples forming, stood on each side of the back garden, which
was mostly lawn.

'Shall we eat outside, Vee, as it's so warm?' Anne gave me
various jobs to do as we went on with our discussion.

'So, Vee,' said Anne, cutting up a tomato. 'Why do you
have to tell them at interview about your illness? Surely it
would make more sense not to.'

'Jim always says that I shouldn't tell, because I might
never be ill again. But if I don't say anything, they're going
to wonder about the gaps in my employment history –
besides which, I have been ill eight times, so there's every
chance of a ninth – and in the end, when I was applying for
jobs, I had to declare it by law. At least that's changed now.
Then quite often there used to be a medical questionnaire.
And in those days, if an employer found out after I'd got the
job, I could be sacked with no redress.'

'Oh, Vee. Damned if you do, damned if you don't. It's
diabolical!'

I told her that there were other things about employers
and their practices which would make her hair curl, but the
most important thing about my life now was that, denied a
job, I had to succumb to the world's attitude and judgement
a second time. What I meant was that, in order to get money
to live on, I had to claim that I was "incapacitated". The
world had won again; everything has to be on *their* terms.
There seemed to be no room for my free will.

We carried our salads and French bread out to the garden
table. A blackbird flew away and sat in a tree at the far end,
plinking his rapid alarm. Anne said she often had a green
woodpecker on the lawn, eating ants. Then she said she felt
sorry for me. She hoped talking to her had helped.

'It is an illness which provokes so many reactions and
emotions and causes untold problems. Do you think you can
sort out your writing now?'

'I think so. Thank you.' I breathed in the fresh, perfumed

air. 'You know, Anne, I spent years of my life trying to fit in. Now, once again, I don't fit in. Somehow, the way I'm seen has become more important than who I am. I'm not going to spend the rest of my life applying for jobs, though. To be rejected non-stop for years would destroy my soul, as would getting a job and then having it taken away again, like Arnold College and then Squaremile. But, you know, one thing I find vaguely amusing – definitely inconsistent – is that I'm still allowed to vote. And another thing: when you get an ordinary doctor's appointment, you're expected to ring if you *can't* make it. But if you have a psychiatric appointment, you're asked to ring if you *can* make it!'

We laughed together.

'So what are you going to do with yourself now?'

'I'll do what I have to do.' I thought I'd better be more specific. 'Write.'

'At least nobody's in a position of authority over you. You've had to give up a lot, but you're probably freer now than you've ever been.'

I had a dream last night. I was alone on a vast beach of flat, wet sand. I felt small and light. The tide was so far out it was a dark blue line against a grey sky and I could only make out a couple of tiny white waves. In the other direction, just as far away, were grass-topped dunes. Then, as I looked straight ahead to where the land curved at the horizon and the blue line of the sea stopped, I saw a black dot, a solitary figure in the distance, walking towards me. I was not afraid; I was calm.

My new neighbours laugh at me now if I go outside, so I spend most of the time indoors. I must revisit the familiar country of the past – finalise the book – before it is too late. I think I know what to do then; the white door stands open. I hope the figure on the beach was Max. He always knows what to do.

Death hath a thousand doors to let out life: I shall find one.
PHILIP MASSINGER

Alone in the attic, Max closed Vee's book. Reading that final chapter, he felt as if he'd lost her all over again. There was an empty space. Then, his arms across the folder on the desk, he began to weep inconsolably. A few moments later, he felt a warm hand squeezing his shoulder.

PART TWO

Amends

23

The Vee Project

The students were back.

"Anyone heard of Maslow's Hierarchy of Needs?" The spotlight is on him.

The student doctors mumble their ignorance.

"I'm not that surprised. It's mostly for psychology students and nurses. But it does help to put things into perspective. Maslow starts with basic human needs, ie food, safety, shelter, warmth and companionship, shown here along the widest part at the bottom, and moves up, like this – " Max is drawing a large triangle on the board and filling in the horizontal strata, writing in the levels of need across it, working his way upwards, "to the pinnacle of achievement for any individual, which Maslow calls 'self-actualisation.' Now the majority of us in Western societies take for granted the fulfilment of the most basic needs. But I think it's important to bear two things in mind: one, the triangular shape implies that not everybody fulfils every need, and two, a person's level of need can change – which is where you and I come in. When a person develops a mental illness, however high their place on this triangle may be, suddenly" – he drops his hand – "the most basic needs become the priority, which is why help is needed."

"Are you saying, then, Dr Greenwood, that someone who is ill cannot reach the pinnacle?" Mr Phillips asks. His light clicks off.

"Not during their illness, no. When they return to normal functioning, they can usually look after their own physical needs, so that the focus shifts to more advanced, even what you might call abstract needs."

"Can you give us an example of this process?" Mr Flint takes his turn.

"Yes. I knew a woman who, when she was well, wrote as a way of finding self-fulfilment. She had food, warmth, clothing etc. in her everyday life and didn't need to worry about these things. But when she became ill, her writing became a series of desperate messages until, in the grip of psychosis, she couldn't write at all. More significantly, nor could she walk, speak, eat or wash herself, so her physical needs became the most important for her survival."

"So when well, she had everything she needed?" Mr Jones has to ask. Click.

"No, that's not what I mean. There were certainly things she did lack when well, but they were not necessarily physical things. Companionship, a relationship perhaps – they were the holes in her triangular cheese, if you like, and it's possible that they contributed to her becoming unwell."

Max knew that, in Maslow's terms, the need for a safe environment was denied to Vee by Sandra . . .

Suddenly there was a crash in the kitchen and Max rushed downstairs to investigate. Helen had her back to him and was crying quietly, her arms stretched out on either side as she gripped the work surface, her head down. On the tiles lay the broken remains of the porcelain dish her mother had bought her.

'Oh, darling. Don't cry! We can replace it.' He picked his way over to her and took her in his arms.

'It's not that, Max . . . ' She was still sobbing. 'I think there must be something wrong with me . . . I keep dropping things and . . . I get pins and needles.'

'Have you got a headache again today?' He had to hide his own anxiety.

'Yes. Well, it comes and goes.'

'Would you like to see the doctor?'

She pulled away from him and crouched down, picking up some larger pieces. 'I don't know. Max, I'll be OK. It's probably nothing. What with work and the business with Jackson, I . . . I'm just tired.'

'If you're sure. Hey, I'll cook tonight. One of my pasta specials, yes? You're on at one, aren't you?'

She nodded. 'Half day, til six.'

'So go up and have a lie down for an hour or so. I'll clear this up.'

She slept for two hours. Max returned to his work in the attic:

"I regarded Sandra as representative of a regime whose darker side was only revealed to me as a consequence of my involvement with Vee, but whose behaviour seemed to be a contributory factor in her death. As a result of this suspicion, I have more than once considered terminating my contract with Squaremile. Then, while Helen was talking about Sandra recently, I realised that things were happening behind the scenes which suggested that the enemy was not the Centre as a whole, but Sandra in particular, who must have hoodwinked the management into following her lead with Vee, and was making the most of her position.

"While this would still prove they didn't care what happened to Vee, it also shows how Sandra could get away with treating her badly. So even if the seniors didn't know exactly what she was doing, as long as she appeared to be ticking all the boxes, they turned a blind eye. Promotion off the house was presumably the management's way of removing Sandra from the front line, as it were, once Vee was out of the picture. Job done. They must have thought highly of her though, to take this expensive route."

Max was too worried about Helen to spend long writing. After waking her at twelve, he went down and ate a sandwich with her.

'Darling, why don't you take a week's leave – they'll just have to manage without you.'

'I can't just drop everything – sorry. I mean, there's too much to do. And don't you want evidence against Sandra? I've had an idea about that. We'll talk it over this evening. I'll be back by seven.'

'Are you sure you're OK to drive?'

'I'll be fine. I've got some painkillers to see me through at work. I'll see you tonight then, Max,' said Helen, putting on her coat and gloves.

'I'm looking forward to hearing this idea.'

She blew him a kiss from the front door.

Back home, Helen seemed fine.

'I found out why I was the one chosen to look after Grove – to go back there, I mean. I had the most experience. Jean is leaving at the end of the week and Sandra's in Portugal until she takes up her new post. She's got two weeks left of her month away; I'd love to know how she wangled a month at once. I can guess, but anyway, they said there was nobody else they could really call on or trust. I do feel a bit used, though, Max. Moved around as it suits them. And I feel . . . trapped. But there's something else, Max.'

He took the few steps from the kitchen to the dining area, with two bowls of pasta, then switched off the television. 'You were saying?'

'Whenever Sandra's been in charge of a house – oh, but hey', she paused to savour the mouthful, 'nice sauce Max. No, but she leaves a trail! Residents' folders get tatty and aren't repaired, the office gets in a mess, some My Life meetings are missed, which reflects badly on the Centre, and shopping trips to get new clothes for some of the people in her care aren't arranged. God alone knows what state Alder was in before the fire. But worst of all, Max,' Helen frowned briefly, 'I had to send two residents to hospital last week. They had been badly neglected. Can you believe it?'

'Yes, actually.'

'Oh, Max. Now I've read her book, I wish I hadn't left Vee on Grove with that woman. I could've picked her to come with me to Birch after the fire, but I had been told to avoid her. I hope I didn't contribute . . . '

'I doubt it. Anyway, why were you told to avoid her?'

'They said . . . '

'Who said?'

'Jack Marshall I think. Yes, he said she was not suitable for further promotion or moving to another house because she was disruptive and kept taking time off sick. I remember now – he tapped the side of his head to show she had mental problems.'

Max's face darkened. 'God, that makes me so angry!'

'Hey, calm down Max. I don't want to get into another ambulance with you. Where's your medication?'

'I'm alright.' He sat back. 'I'm more worried about you. How have you been today, in yourself?'

'Not too bad.' Helen cleared away the pasta dishes and fetched two yoghurts. 'Vanilla or strawberry?'

'Vanilla please. Come on then, my love, I'm itching to know what your idea is!'

She took a deep breath, and announced that they should prepare a document, a report, covering the goings-on in Grove as well as Vee's treatment. Then they could present it to senior management. They both knew that she was in the perfect position.

'I think that's a brilliant idea! In fact, I think it's really the only way forward!'

So gripped were they by the excitement of having a definite plan that they stayed at the table for the rest of the evening discussing strategy. Max was interested in what the junior staff might have to say, like a fly on the wall. Helen had already thought of this and was planning to talk to them individually, and tape them. With their consent, of course, and anonymously, because any methods she and Max used must be beyond reproach. Max could see problems with this; for example the first one might talk about it to the others. Again, Helen countered this by saying that she had got to know these people, so knew who got on with whom and who was likely to cause trouble; based on this, she had already decided who the first person would be.

Max would still be at the Centre on Tuesday mornings if Helen needed him urgently, but they soon got into a routine. When she was on earlies, she would report back in the evening any developments concerning Sandra or Grove. If she was on a late shift, Max would spend the evening keeping up with the notes for the report and beginning to put it together. He kept a close watch on Helen to make sure she didn't get too stressed. He was also secretly planning the holiday they would have earned, somewhere nice and warm, which would lift her spirits when this was all over.

They knew that their actions could have an impact on the lives of others. Max thought those two weeks before Sandra's return would be enough to get the information they needed and interview the juniors so they could present the report to the Chief Executive. Better go straight to the top, bypassing Jack Marshall, they thought. Nevertheless, it was possible that the management had moved Helen to Grove for a purpose not dissimilar to theirs, so perhaps Max and Helen would have Jack Marshall's support, especially if he was impressed by Helen's improvements, and even if he didn't know the true motives behind her activities or enquiries. Max recognised, however, that it was important to keep an open mind about the people they were dealing with: in his view, assumptions of any kind were among the most dangerous lapses of mankind, made by those who think they're observant.

For the whole of that first week, Max and Helen devoted their energies to the Vee Project. Not only did Max have the report to prepare, but he also had to write up the discussions he had with Helen. On the second day, he wrote the last piece about Vee herself:

"A textbook definition of prejudice is seen in the way Sandra despised Vee for something she couldn't help. Sandra was the last straw for Vee, the last link in a long chain. Vee grew up with the idea that mental illness was a sign of weakness, then one day she found herself diagnosed with bipolar disorder. Despite the catastrophic effects of this, she retained insight, enough to record what she felt, and she recognised that she was not alone. When she saw those long-stay patients in West Pluting, she was, I think, humbled: they were worse off than she was.

"But I think the most significant effect of her illness was that people started treating her differently. Before diagnosis, she hadn't needed to prove anything. She just lived; nobody requires a certificate of sanity. Things that had once been easy for her, like getting a job, were suddenly much more difficult, if not impossible. She had to start proving herself now, and there was no script. She encountered stigma and negative assumptions at every turn, even when she got a job at Squaremile. There, she began by assuming, as one might in such a setting, that people were going to be sympathetic. Instead, she had disciplinary hearings and warnings and in the end was sacked because Sandra thought it her duty to discriminate. If you feel that others are suspicious of you, the tendency is to feel guilty."

Liz was first on the list of junior staff who had to be called over from Birch. As Helen had said, when she had taken up the reins in Birch after Bill's death, she had got to know the different personalities on the staff. She knew Liz to be a bit of a loner, unlikely to say much about what went on today. Helen brought in coffee, and invited Liz to sit down opposite her, so that her face was lit by the window. This was an old trick Max had taught Helen. She tried to make sure they weren't disturbed. She described Liz as being about twenty, of mixed race, with large dark eyes. Helen played Max the first part of the recording, which they would have to edit because of the name.

"'I've called you in, Liz, to see how you think things are going. Do you like working on the Centre?'

'Yeah, pretty much.' Her voice was quite deep.

'Is there anything you want to say about your working conditions?'

'Don't fink so.'

'Now, I want to check if you mind me taping our chat. You can refuse. The tape will only be played to senior staff and nothing you say will be held against you, because it will be anonymous. Your name won't appear. So you can say what you really think, and when the tape has served its purpose, it will be wiped, OK?'

'I don't mind. Got nuffink to 'ide.'"

Helen proceeded to play the whole interview at home that night. It confirmed what they knew about about Sandra to a certain extent, despite the fact that Liz presented a simplified version. But they needed more. Helen decided she would speak to Sue, Sally and Brian next; they had known Sandra on Alder before the fire. Last of all would come Nat, when she came back from her week's leave. She would have been last in any case, with good reason: she would be the most likely to cause trouble. That said, she would also be the most likely to provide good evidence. Meanwhile Jack Marshall, fresh from his management update course, was interviewing candidates for the manager's post on Grove where Helen was locum; a new manager had taken over in Birch.

Helen desperately wanted to get back to her original house, Sycamore. She had put a good deal of effort into improving the systems, and morale, both on Grove and Birch, and her enthusiasm was now beginning to wane. She would come home with horror stories about the residents and Max could see that the job was taking it out of her. She really should see a doctor; her headaches and tiredness continued to worry Max.

At the end of the first week, as they sat at the table again after dinner, Helen told Max how Nat had come into the office, her long, dyed blond hair flowing loose. She was wearing make-up, earrings and a chain round her neck, and she had rings on three fingers of each hand. Helen repeated their conversation, putting on a convincing accent for Nat.

'I said to her, "Before we start, Nat, I want to remind you of what I said before: those rings are unhygienic, given the work we do. And you should tie your hair back. If it got caught in the hoist or something, you'd know about it."'

Max nodded and found himself smiling with anticipation.

'Nat sniffed, and chewed. "Sandra and Jean didn't mind", she said.'

He laughed at the intonation.

'Then I said, "Well I'm Helen, and I do mind. Besides

which, it's not just me being awkward. It's a Health and Safety issue."'

'You old schoolma'am!' Max blurted out, teasing.

Helen looked at him across the debris of their meal. 'But it's true, Max!'

'Oh, I know that. So what happened next?'

'Well, I realised this wasn't a good start if I wanted Nat's co-operation, so I got her to tell me about herself and what she thought she'd achieved at Squaremile. And I congratulated her on her promotion.'

'You buttered her up, you mean.'

'I did. I'm not proud! But at least then I was able to reintroduce the idea of a taped conversation. And I got what I wanted.'

By the end of the following evening, Max had finished transcribing Liz's and Nat's interviews. They would be ready if required. The other recordings Helen had made in between, during the week, turned out to be unusable for one reason or another, although they gave Helen a certain amount of information. Helen had been shocked and angered by Nat's complacency. Vee was dead, after all, and Nat could only snigger when she was mentioned. Max too was disappointed by the attitude of the juniors, although Liz's attitude was not as destructive as Nat's.

On a more positive note, however, Max and Helen were pleased by the fact that the recordings would provide the evidence they needed, excellent ammunition for what lay ahead. They knew that very soon they would have to round off the report and approach someone with a view to organising a meeting.

Sandra was due back in a week, on Thursday. They decided to start by going to Jack Marshall in the end, as he was Helen's line manager and Max thought they should follow protocol after all. The Friday before, she tried to see Jack, but he proved elusive and then had the weekend off. Max knew Helen didn't like Jack, but he wasn't sure why. At last she was able to make an appointment with his secretary for Tuesday at 11 a.m. in his office. She asked if Max could also be present. He had one patient at ten, then he was free until 2 p.m. But Jack's secretary would not agree to it, even though Helen claimed she needed the moral support of her husband. According to the secretary, it was strictly Squaremile business; a psychiatrist was not thought necessary.

24

Dr Conway

Max noticed that the combination of seeing Jack Marshall and Sandra's imminent return made Helen more than usually anxious. She focused on her appearance, despite her exhaustion. The day before, Max had gone to Vee's inquest, which was pretty wearing, then he had worked on the Vee report and his own notes late into the night. But at the moment, Helen was obviously in need of reassurance.

'Max, you don't think this top is too low-cut, do you?'

'You look fine, darling, as always. I just wish I could be there to see Jack with you, but it'll be OK; there's no need to worry.'

Helen gave Max her helpless child look and he wondered what kind of man Jack was to inspire such apparent fear. Max drove her to Squaremile. It made sense to use one car when they were both in on a Tuesday, even though it meant he had about an hour and a half before his first appointment. He parked round the back of the Day Hospital and staff lounge, where there was some outdoor seating.

He sat on one of the worn leatherette benches in the staff lounge with a coffee. This lounge must be due for a facelift, he thought, as he noticed the ubiquitous magnolia was peeling round the doorframes and under the windowsills. A group of metal-framed chairs had been arranged round each of the two large tables, one at each end of the room. The black padded built-in seating stretched in two arcs under the windows, giving the impression of eyebrows, with the tables as eyes. These were the meanderings of a tired mind. There *were* other tables and chairs, next to other windows. Where the bridge of the nose would be, to his left, stood a huge plant resembling a palm. But what had once been considered good design was now shabby and in need of some tlc. Max was alone except for the bar staff, clattering crockery and cutlery.

A length of brown carpet, sunk into the floor, extended from the admin. block offices at one end to the Day Hospital at the other, dividing the seating area from the bar. The office he borrowed every week was the first on the right in the Hospital.

Jack Marshall appeared, heading towards the admin. offices. Max had only met him once, briefly, before today. They were about the same age, but Jack still had a full head of hair, which is more than Max could say, and a lean physique, suggesting he had once been a runner. His bearing was such that Max guessed he had been in the Forces. Max stood up.

'Ah, Dr Greenwood. I'm seeing your wife this morning.' His Birmingham accent hadn't registered last time, but this was their first proper conversation.

'That's right,' said Max.

'She's a very attractive woman,' he smiled. 'You should be careful!'

Max smiled back. 'I know. I'm a lucky man.'

Jack went on his way. Max decided to go next door, to the borrowed office, to do some paperwork, but he was preoccupied with the Project and his concern over Helen. His desk was under the window, and a movement outside caught his attention. A little way off, Jack Marshall was talking to a woman in her late forties or so, with short fair hair, whose body language was very controlled; no doubt she was aware that people might be watching. Then Jack raised his arm to indicate that they should go indoors. Max moved aside quickly as they approached the entrance to the right of his window. He could hear their voices but couldn't make out any words. They went through the staff lounge to Jack's office and Max eased across in his seat.

He realised it was time for his patient, and looked up just as she was arriving with a care assistant. Half an hour later, after arranging a follow-up appointment, the care assistant wheeled her away. Max came out of the office as the woman he had seen outside with Jack was making her way back along the brown carpet, still talking to him.

'I know it's not good, Sandra, but you'll have to tell them – .'

'– Oh, look, Jack, they won't say anything . . . '

'Hello again, Dr Greenwood.' With a nervous laugh, Jack interrupted what was clearly a very private conversation. 'Have you met our Health and Safety Officer, Sandra Wheatley?'

Sandra smiled. 'You must be our weekly psychiatrist.'

'That's right. Well, I'd better be on my way, if you'll excuse me.'

Helen had decided she should see her GP, without telling Max. Her appointment was at 11.30, after Jack. Having brought the spare car keys, she drove the three miles to the village, hoping she would be back in time to meet up with Max for lunch.

Dr Conway was a small, dapper man of about forty, his jet black hair brushed with grey at the temples. Dark, intelligent eyes shone from under his thick brows.

'Hello, Mrs Greenwood. Take a seat. We don't see you in here very often! What can I do for you today?'

'I'm a bit worried.' To her surprise, she found it difficult to admit she had a problem, now she had the chance to do so. She had always been fairly healthy and far more concerned with helping other people through *their* difficult times and health problems. 'I've been having terrible headaches.'

'How often?'

'They're getting more frequent – nearly every day, or part of a day now, in fact.'

'And when did they start?' Dr Conway sat back in his chair, watching her and listening intently.

'Oh, about two months ago, I suppose.'

'What does your husband think? Did he get you to come here?' He chuckled. 'I know what health professionals are like when it comes to seeing doctors.'

'He doesn't know. That is, he knows I get headaches, but not how bad they are. So far I've managed to control myself so that . . . He doesn't know I'm seeing you today, although I think he might be starting to get worried.'

'Are the headaches worse in the morning, or later in the day?'

'Oh, first thing in the morning, there's no doubt! I have to have painkillers ready by the bed or I can't get up.'

'Do you have any other symptoms?'

'Such as?'

'Dizziness, clumsiness, ataxia, nausea, for example?'

'I have noticed that I'm more clumsy lately. I keep dropping things, spilling drinks, that kind of thing. I keep getting pins and needles in my right hand. Max won't let me wash up nowadays. And some days I have to take an afternoon nap, which I never used to do. My eyes just won't stay open if I'm not at work.'

'Right. I see.' Dr Conway glanced at the reference books on the shelf above his desk.

'What do you think it is, doctor?'

'There are a few possibilities. Is there any hereditary illness in your family?'

'Not that I know of. Can I ask . . . ?'

'Go on.'

'Is there something wrong with my brain? Like a tumour or something?'

'Hmm. We can't rule it out. I'm going to refer you for tests, including an MRI scan. In the meantime, I'll prescribe you a stronger painkiller.'

'Thank you.'

He printed off the prescription and filled in a form.

'Here. Have the blood test today – the nurse should still be there.' Helen made to get up, but he went on: 'Before you go, Mrs Greenwood, I'd like to make two recommendations. One, that you don't drive and two, that you talk to your husband. The one will necessitate the other. But things would be made easier anyway if you discuss it at this stage.'

'Rather than wait for some worse news, you mean?'

'Well, yes. But more importantly, he is your husband. I'm assuming that your relationship is good?'

'We're fine.'

'Well, he's there to support you. You don't have to deal with everything on your own. He would come to you if he had a problem, wouldn't he?'

'I expect so. But you make it sound so easy!'

'OK. You can drive back up to the Centre, but not after that. Come and see me again when you've had the tests: the scan appointment should come through quite quickly, and we'll take it from there.'

Luckily she was able to park the car in the same space, although there was still the chance Max had missed her. It was a blustery day at the end of March, sun alternating rapidly with cloud. One moment the café tables nearby were gleaming, too bright to look at, the next they were a dull grey. Groups of people came and went. Max and Helen, meeting for lunch, sat indoors by the window with their trays.

'You're miles away!' said Helen. 'Don't you want to know, then, how it went with Jack?' She had given him the chance to ask, but now his time was up.

'Sorry dear. How did it go?' Max felt a surge of excitement, in spite of everything.

'It was . . . interesting.' She looked left and right. 'I don't want to go into too much detail here, but he said . . . ' She waited for a screaming child to be taken out, then watched Max unwrap his sandwiches. She said she couldn't face anything to eat. She leant forward, confidentially. 'Jack said he had every confidence in Sandra, even though he admitted there had been one or two complaints from other staff which is why, he says, she was moved off the house. I said I wondered why Sandra hadn't been demoted or disciplined, rather than promoted.'

'How did he respond to that?'

'He wasn't prepared to explain; he just said there were other issues involved.'

'But I thought you were going to try and arrange a proper hearing, for our report.'

'I was, but other things got in the way.'

'What about Vee? Did you talk about her?'

'He maintains Sandra did all she could to help her – .'

'– I can't understand it!'

'Sssshh! Keep it down Max!'

Max tried to control himself, managing not to thump the table. 'But it's staring him in the face! The woman should be sacked!'

'I know that, you know that, but Jack Marshall knows something else.' Helen looked annoyed.

'Helen, I met Sandra today.'

'What! She's not due back at work until Thursday.'

'She came in to see Jack, and it seemed like an urgent discussion.'

'Huh, getting their stories straight, I expect.' Helen stared out into the sunlight.

'Sorry . . . have I missed something here? What do you mean by that?'

'Oh Max! You're such an innocent! Don't you realise they're having an affair?

Jack's known for, well . . . '

'Ah. That would explain a lot.' Max paused, embarrassed.

Helen leant over again, whispering, delighting in the scandal. 'I must tell you this! I practically caught them *at it* one day in Alder office! When I went into the house it was quiet as the grave. I knocked on the office door and suddenly I heard a lot of movement within, and Sandra's flustered voice saying something like: "Yes, that'll be fine, thanks Jack. Come in!" I had to smile. Anyway, Max, that's the reason I didn't want to hand the report over to Jack in the first place, or arrange the big meeting through him.' Helen sat back in her seat and spoke normally. 'We'll take it to the top, OK?'

They were able to get an initial appointment with the Chief Executive a week later. But Max wanted to know why Helen refused to drive anywhere. Saying she didn't feel well was enough for the first couple of times, but then Max began to get worried. She realised she couldn't prolong his agony and had to come clean. He gave her the chance.

'Helen, I came to find you after I'd seen my patient on Tuesday, but you weren't in the House and the car had gone. Where were you?'

'I had an appointment with my GP. Come for a walk with me, Max, your favourite walk. We can get to the far end and back before it's dark now.'

But in the middle of putting on her boots, she was suddenly overwhelmed. Tears burned her eyes; the whole story came out. Max took her in his arms and held her for a long time.

25

Dick Montgomery

Dick Montgomery's secretary opened the door to his office. Brigadier Richard Montgomery, who was in his sixties, made himself comfortable in his large leather chair. He wore a tailored suit and spoke with a cut-glass accent. His bearing, like that of Jack Marshall, betrayed his military background, but this time there was definitely the added ingredient of public school. His tie bore an unusual symbol. Helen, once again without Max, sat in an ordinary chair.

'You say you have a complaint about a member of the senior management, Sandra Wheatley.'

'My husband and I have prepared a report, Mr Montgomery,' said Helen, placing a copy of the document, in its red cover, on the desk in front of him. She went on, a little less confidently, as Dick had not yet reacted to the report. 'It gives examples of Sandra's conduct and we think it deserves your attention.'

There was a pause, during which Dick Montgomery picked up a fountain pen and breathed heavily once or twice, apparently deep in thought. Helen thought he had an air of sadness which he was trying to conceal.

'Why did you come to me first with this and not to Mr Marshall?'

'I did see him first, but the questions raised are sufficiently serious to bring the matter to you myself, rather than wait indefinitely for "procedure" to take its course.'

'And can you tell me what, precisely, is your husband's involvement in this affair? He is not a full-time employee here, after all.'

'Sir, Vee Gates, who used to work here, was his patient.

He has evidence to suggest that Sandra's attitude towards her was a contributory factor in Vee's suicide.'

'Ha, ha! Really?' Dick coughed. 'You expect me to believe that a respected member of my staff had something to do with *that*? How is that possible, Mrs Greenwood?'

'We *do* want you to believe it, yes.' Helen was fired up now and her Scots accent was in evidence. 'Because it's true. And that's not all. When she was House Manager, Sandra was not really, well, managing. As you may know, I have just spent some time on Grove – .'

'– Are you saying now that Ms Wheatley is incompetent, as well as driving people to suicide?' Dick chuckled complacently and shook his head. He put down his pen and, his elbows on the desk, tapped his fingertips together.

'We need you to take this seriously, sir,' Helen asserted. 'There are residents on Grove who appear to have been neglected.'

'Now we have the dreaded word "neglect" as well. What will it be next, mass slaughter that nobody's witnessed except you?'

'With respect, sir, I don't think you're giving me a fair hearing.' Helen's annoyance was beginning to show. 'Everybody would love to think that an organisation like this ran smoothly all the time, but the fact is that where there are people, there will be mistakes. I think you should read the report in full and make a few enquiries of your own before laughing us out of court.'

'You're wrong.' Dick Montgomery leant forward and peered over his glasses at Helen like an ageing headmaster. 'I do take these things seriously, Mrs Greenwood. And I intend to be fair. But you must admit these are pretty grave accusations. The Centre has been running successfully for over seventy years. I need to understand why, when you two come along, problems like this come to light. Now,' He stood up. 'I will read your report and I will see you again in a week's time. On that occasion, I will invite Jack Marshall, Sandra Wheatley and a representative from the union to be present. Your husband will be there too, yes? We shall hold a formal hearing in the boardroom next door. After all, I think we're still civilised enough to allow Ms Wheatley the chance to defend herself, wouldn't you say?'

26

The Girls

Helen hoped that those who followed her in charge of Birch and Grove would appreciate her hard work, but she knew that efficiency can be taken for granted. Grove would have its new manager in the next day or so, according to the grapevine. She was forcing herself to keep going in the meantime; the fear of not getting everything done meant she felt the need to organise Max too.

'Have you rescheduled your Tuesday appointments?'

'All taken care of. Hey! I'm worried about the meeting too, on top of everything else, but we . . . ' He reached across the table and took both her hands in his. 'We have to get through this, stay focused, together.' Their eyes met. 'And we've got Grace and Anna coming at the weekend, haven't we? You'll see your girls.' He let her get on with her meal, but he had to admit he was having difficulty finishing his lasagne, even if it was home made. 'The hardest part's done now the report's sent out. Thank goodness for that at least!'

'I wonder what Monty makes of it. Oh, I forgot to tell you that I've asked that someone from Social Services be present next week, because of the neglect, you know. And for moral support, really . . . I faxed them the report as well.'

'Right. No more shop-talk now', said Max. 'Let's go for that walk we were going to have the other day.' They abandoned the kitchen.

'I can see why you like that walk so much, Max,' Helen said as she struggled out of her boots, back in the porch afterwards. 'Can you pass me some newspaper? And now spring's arrived, there are loads of birds!'

'They're all looking for a mate. I'm lucky, I didn't have to sing to get mine!' Max laughed, realising it was the first time he'd done so for a while.

'Phew! I'm glad I'm not a bird then! Narrow escape, that.' Helen flung her arms round him.

'How are you feeling today, darling?' he asked, wanting to keep hold of her.

'Not too bad. It comes and goes. It's horrible not being able to drive, though. Perhaps Dr Conway was worried I'd have a fit or something. I don't know.' She broke free, not having the time to allow emotions to surface.

Max smiled. 'What shall we do for the girls, then?'

This was always Vee's worst time of year. "You'll know what to do", she had said. So Max had to make sure he did. In St Peter's churchyard, he knelt down, trying to tidy up a bit. Then he placed a pot of primulas next to her stone. He must have said something out loud, because the next moment, a familiar voice said calmly: 'Who's that then, Max?'

He was caught off guard by his former colleague. 'Oh, hello Sue. You made me jump! This is – a friend.'

She read Vee's inscription but it obviously meant nothing to her. 'My dad is just down there. I come here about once a fortnight.'

It was strangely refreshing to be able to talk shop for a few minutes, although he needed to get back home, not just for Helen and the Vee Project, but because he had a nagging feeling about Sandra.

'Fancy a drink?'

'Another time, thanks Sue.'

Max realised he had overlooked something. When Vee started having disciplinary hearings and when they put verbal warnings on her file, Sandra had not been involved. She couldn't have been: Vee was still working in Forest House. She and Sandra had not even met then. This led him to consider a more sinister possibility. Sandra's role would still be to make life as unpleasant as possible for Vee, yes, but what if she wasn't pulling the strings? So who was then? This made sense: Sandra was a good choice of protagonist, given her prejudice, and Vee was put in Alder House for a reason; she was a thorn in Squaremile's side. With the lure of promotion, Sandra could give full vent to her spite to make sure Vee left. Of course the management could not have anticipated her suicide, but it was clear they'd closed ranks. There was just one thing Sandra could not see: she would be a convenient scapegoat if her behaviour was questioned.

He had to put this to Helen before Tuesday. Today was Friday. Sunday was Helen's birthday. The girls were coming tomorrow. It would have to be tonight. If a social worker was coming to the meeting, at least they wouldn't be outnumbered, but in that connection, he had to make an urgent phone call. When Helen came home at six o'clock, he explained his ideas.

'I think you're right', said Helen. 'But does it make that much difference in the end?'

'Yes, because it means we can't rely on anyone. But don't worry. We'll show them.'

'Max, where's the report?'

'Oh it's here somewhere.'

'I want to read it through again before we need it.'

They kept everything to do with the report at home to avoid prying eyes, and never let one word slip about it at work. He sat at his computer and declined the offer of a cup of coffee. He too was finding it a real effort to concentrate; it was no longer an act of escapism to write his notes. The student doctors had packed up and gone home. Recent developments had to be recorded accurately and the stage set for Tuesday. Things were moving. Helen looked over his shoulder and he had to remind her that she was not allowed to read any of his own work yet.

Is it in this pile?'

'What?'

'The report!'

'Helen, do you have to have it right this minute?'

She looked at him, surprised. 'No, I s'pose it can wait. Max, are you OK?'

'I'll be fine. Look, I'm sorry. This whole thing must be getting to me. I didn't mean to snap at you. It's there, look, where you left it.'

'Max . . . I don't think I can go through with this.' Her words landed like a bomb.

'But . . . are you sure?' Max spoke quietly now, remembering her situation. 'Only we've worked so hard to get this far . . . and it's all set up. I won't be able to do it on my own.'

He moved away from the computer and put his hands over his face. He felt old and tired, they were both trying to do too much, Helen might be seriously ill and he kept seeing Vee. Sunset and champagne. He was struggling.

'Vee's not around any more, is she?' he said, leaning against the desk. 'She can't do this. You said you'd help me, try and put things right. People who find themselves in Vee's position in the future will thank you if you can just hold on. Please, darling.'

She knew he was right, but knowing that didn't suddenly make her feel better. He knew he had to change the subject. He tried to smile. 'Bet you're looking forward to this afternoon, though, aren't you?'

'Yes! Grace said she'd be here about three but Anna wasn't quite sure.'

'Helen?' He looked up.

'Yes?'

'I'll let you decide if you want to tell the girls today, but they'll have to know soon, won't they? Think about it. Now come here.' He stood up and stretched out his arms.

They embraced silently. Her hair smelt good. 'I love you, Mrs Greenwood.'

Anna arrived about two hours after Grace and they spent the evening talking, laughing and eating. Helen was more relaxed than he'd seen her for a while; he put this down partly to the relief she felt at the prospect of being back in charge of Sycamore soon (her deputy would probably be grateful too), and also to the presence of her clever girls. He just hoped she wasn't over-compensating.

'Hey girls!' she exclaimed at the table; 'You've both got too thin. Come on, you need some proper food. I remember what it was like to be a student.'

'Did you meet any dinosaurs?' Anna laughed.

'Less of that, thank you!'

'Mind you, some of our professors – I reckon they dust them off each day when they bring them out of the cupboard!' Anna helped herself to more vegetables.

'Tell us about Oxford again, Dad.' Two years older than her sister, Grace had always been the quiet, studious one. Her finals were approaching.

'I shouldn't think there's much difference in university life wherever you go', replied Max. 'It's what you make of the experience that counts. You have to strike a balance between working and having fun. But you know all this; I've said it before.'

'Yes, but what Grace meant was, tell us again what you got up to as medical students!' Anna smiled with mischief in her eyes and nudged her sister.

'Oh, no!' Max exclaimed. 'That's off-limits, especially while we're eating!' Everybody roared with laughter.

Later, Helen was about to open the kitchen door when she overheard Anna talking to her father as they prepared to wash up.

'She doesn't look well, Dad,' she said quietly. 'She seemed to be putting on a jolly act just now for our benefit, but she's pale and . . . I was shocked by the look in her eyes. Is she in pain? What's wrong with her?'

'Oh, she's been overdoing it lately. The truth is . . . we need that holiday, but we're working on a special project right now and we're determined to see it through. You know what your mother's like.'

'Am I allowed to know what it is?'

Just then, Helen heard Grace coming behind her with a load of crockery, so she went in first.

'I see Dad's given you the rest of the night off,' Grace said to her mother, as Anna cleared some space. 'You should make the most of it.'

Sunday came and with it gifts for Helen. The girls brought their parents breakfast in bed, complete with a single red rose in a vase. They sang "Happy Birthday" as they came in, then left them to it. Dr Conway's painkillers were now only slightly more effective than the old ones, but at least these days Helen didn't have to hide what she was doing from Max. When Grace and Anna returned, each held a small parcel and card.

'Hope you like this, Mum,' said Anna. It was what they call a "vest" nowadays: a sleeveless sun-top.

'It'll be lovely for hot days. Thank you, darling. And what's this? French recipes. Ah, thank you Grace.'

'Talking of which,' said Max, 'we're going to Lisette's for Sunday lunch, so we'd better start getting ready. Oh, and one other thing – I've paid for your present, Helen, but it won't be delivered until August.'

'Oh, I see. Aah! I see! At least I think, hope, I do!' She leant over and kissed him sharply and loudly. Both girls were smiling; Max had told them about this present when they wanted to know what to buy for their mother, but had sworn them to secrecy.

'I'm assuming,' Helen went on, in a rising intonation, 'that the vest might come in particularly useful in connection with this mysterious gift?'

'I'm not saying any more.' Max dramatised his reply. 'I know we're not supposed to keep things from each other, but – ' then he spoke in his normal tone, 'I'm making an exception in this case.'

Helen laughed.

One of Bach's Brandenburg Concertos was playing quietly as they entered Lisette's. Their coats were taken away.

'Ah, Dr Grainwood. 'ow nass to see you egen!' They were shown to a large, oval table next to the window and the waiter who recognised Max checked they were comfortable and gave them their menus. 'An' zees must be your waf: 'appy birsday, Madame! Are zeez your dotteurs?'

'Yes, thank you!'

'But Madame does not look old eneurf!'

Helen beamed at him. The table was beautiful, decorated with green and white flowers on a white damask cloth. The cutlery caught the light. Max whispered, 'Happy Birthday darling', in Helen's ear, then announced, 'Have whatever you like, ladies!'

It was a different experience for Helen to come here in daylight. In the evening at one time there used to be candles on every table, until they were deemed a fire hazard. The soft light would flash on the waiter's cufflinks as he poured the wine. She didn't know why, but when they poured wine in a restaurant, it always sounded more inviting than when it was poured at home. When the waiter moved away, the only thing visible would be his white sleeves. Helen recalled Max's farewell dinner here with Chris and Sue. From time to time a door at the back of the room would open, allowing delicious smells to escape; then it would swing shut again with scarcely a sound. Today, she could see this door beyond the other tables. It was painted black, for the evening effect, and the surrounding decor was also dark. Now her head was pounding again, clamping her brain. She recalled Vee's description of the black corridors in her mind . . .

'Helen!' Max was staring at her.

'Sorry. Miles away.' She fiddled with her bag, then put it on the floor. They ordered.

'What's everyone having to drink then?' asked Max.

The conversation dealt with driving lessons for Grace after her exams, the accidents her mother and father had had, and what was currently regarded as a "good" car.

'What about greenhouse gases?' said Anna. 'Everybody's worried about pollution, but most people just carry on as if cars make no difference.'

'Can't save it for the debating society, then?' Grace pretended to be annoyed.

'Yes, actually.' Anna was sometimes sharp, not out of

anger, but from a desire to proceed with what she wanted to say. 'But Dad, this is serious. The planet is dying. We're so wrapped up in our own little worlds, each of us, that we forget we depend on this *one* world for our very survival.'

The family fell silent. Max gave his daughter a look which said, "Not now, Anna." He winked at Helen. 'Everyone got something in their glasses? Good. Here's to a wonderful wife and mother!'

'You're not having any wine, Mum?' Grace was surprised.

'Thought I'd give it a rest.' She had to take some more painkillers, urgently.

'But it's your birthday! You usually have a drink when you're out. There's nothing wrong, is there? Are you on antibiotics or something?' Grace was like a dog with a bone.

'No, nothing like that. Just didn't want any.' Helen knew this wasn't convincing, and she caught Max's eye as he tried to finish his pâté.

The rest of the meal passed without further embarrassment and Helen managed to get to the ladies to take her pills. The girls left together for the station that evening and the house was suddenly quiet.

'Don't worry, Helen.' Max tried to console her, knowing the sadness in her silence. He washed up some cups. 'It won't be long before we see Grace again. Her Finals aren't far off, so she'll be busy . . . ' he put his hands on Helen's shoulders and could feel the tension.

'I *will* tell them,' she said, 'when I get the chance and when I know more about it.' She picked up a tea towel.

'Then we'll have a graduation to go to – and something nice after that to look forward to.'

'Oh, Max. Thank you for a lovely birthday. But I never miss those girls as much as when they've just left.'

'Look, I know you're tired darling. You didn't eat much, either. Why don't you have an early night?' He turned to face her. 'When is your scan?'

'It's on Wednesday. And I've decided to keep going with our project. I must.'

Max grabbed the tea towel, threw it aside, and embraced and kissed her. 'I can see where Anna gets it from.'

'There's one thing I need to do first. I need to see my Mum. I haven't seen her for about three months, except for that concert, but everything was alright then.'

26

The Boardroom (1)

The room was full of morning sunlight. Dick Montgomery, resplendent in light grey suit, white shirt and royal blue bow tie and handkerchief, was at the head of the table, flanked by Sandra and Jack: a Squaremile triumvirate under the window. Along the table was a row of water jugs and glasses and as each person took a seat, a copy of the report in its red cover would appear in front of them among their papers. On Sandra's right sat a lady in her thirties with intricately braided hair, and at a separate small table just behind and to the right of Dick Montgomery sat his secretary.

Helen and Max walked in.

'Ah, do sit down,' said the Chief Executive. Max and Helen sat on opposite sides: he was next to Jack, on Dick's left, facing the lady they didn't know.

'You have invited somebody from Social Services, Mrs Greenwood. Is he or she coming?' Dick raised his eyebrows at her and tapped his pen lightly on the table.

'I hope so.' Helen was not particularly worried, although she had no idea who was coming. Max knew.

Dick looked ostentatiously at his watch. 'We shall have to start soon.' He probably had plans for lunch at some club. Then the door was pushed open and a briefcase appeared, followed by its owner, a tall man in his forties who was slightly out of breath. Max had phoned to ask for him specifically, and nobody else, and again to make sure the faxed report had reached him.

'Sorry I'm a bit late,' the man said. 'Traffic.' He decided to sit next to Helen, by the door. She gave Max a look of muted surprise.

'We were just about to begin,' said Dick. 'Our esteemed Director of Care has been unavoidably detained, I'm afraid. He sends his apologies, but I'm sure we'll be able to manage without him. Now, do we all know each other? This is Jack Marshall . . . ' He went round the table. ' . . . This is Janice Olubi, from Union HQ – and what is your name, please, social worker?'

'Jim Gates, sir.'

Dick Montgomery was having the "headmaster effect" all over again.

'And I'm a Care Manager,' Jim added, carefully correcting Dick. Max tried to avoid eye contact with Jim.

'I see, I see. Gates . . . why is that name familiar to me?' Dick paused. No answer was forthcoming, as nobody wanted to cause Dick embarrassment. 'Anyway, we have a lot to discuss, so let us proceed. You all received a copy of the agenda, I trust?'

Everyone murmured and, rustling, put the piece of paper on top of the report.

'As you can see, we have two main items: one, the issue of whether or not there has been neglect of residents in our care and two, whether the Centre discriminated against Ms Victoria Gates, member of st – ah! That's where I've heard the name!'

Dick Montgomery put down his paper slowly, folded his hands so that the thumbs protruded at the top and peered at Jim over his glasses. 'Bit of a coincidence, wouldn't you say? Are you related to Ms Gates, Mr Gates?'

Jim stayed calm. 'Yes, sir. She was my sister.'

'Ah, now,' said Dick, leaning forward. 'I don't think this is in the book. What do you think – Dr Greenwood, Ms Olubi?'

'It is not usual practice,' said Ms Olubi, with her Nigerian intonation. 'And I find it strange that it should be Mr Gates when it could have been anybody.'

'Good point, my dear, good point.' He paused. 'Can you cast any light on this, Dr Greenwood?'

Helen narrowed her eyes at Max across the table in the

heavy pause which followed. It was the sort meant for confessions.

'Sir. I take full responsibility. I contacted Jim directly. It is his sister we're talking about, after all, and I thought he – .'

'– I wanted to find out what happened to Vee here,' Jim interrupted, to Max's relief. He went on: 'I wanted to know what went wrong, who was involved, why, and I wanted some kind of closure. I was glad Dr Greenwood got in touch.'

There was another pause. Dick began fiddling with his pen again. He looked at each person in turn. Then he threw himself back in his chair and dropped the pen on the folder.

'Well? What shall we do?' He put his hands behind his head.

'Sir,' said Helen, 'we need a care manager to be present for Item 1, if nothing else – the neglect.'

'Alleged neglect,' Dick replied.

Helen continued, 'But the point is, if we don't let Jim stay, we'll have to postpone the meeting.'

'That is a valid observation, Mrs Greenwood. How do the rest of you feel?' Dick looked at his watch again.

'Oh, let's just get on with it, shall we?' Sandra was impatient. 'Some of us have more important things to do than sit around here all day.'

'Right then,' Dick went on. 'Are we all agreed that Mr Gates should stay?' There were nods and murmurs. 'I'll take that as a yes. So, we will break for coffee at eleven. The staff lounge is at your disposal and now let's press on with Item 1. You have all read the report produced by Mrs Greenwood?' Again there was a murmur of assent.

'Point of order, Mr Montgomery.' Max raised his hand; Dick seemed to have made a huge assumption. 'Since it is the Centre which is, so to speak, in the dock, is it right that *you* chair the meeting?'

'Oh, we're not going to have all that voting nonsense, on top of everything else, are we?' Dick was exasperated. He held onto the table as if he would rather leave.

'I don't think that will be necessary, but I do think it

would be more appropriate if someone else, who is not directly involved with the Centre, were to take the chair.'

'In other words, you, Dr Greenwood.'

Max felt his hands sweating. 'But only if everyone is happy with that. For the sake of objectivity. As far as we . . . can.'

Dick gave a heavy sigh and continued wearily, speaking in the rather childish, heavy rhythm of someone who will never accept that another person knows better and who assumes that every delay is meant personally: 'Does anybody object to Dr Greenwood chairing this meeting?' Nobody spoke. '*Please* can we get on then? Over to you. Although I still can't really understand why I'm allowing you to be present, let alone Mr Gates.' He looked at Max, his mouth taut, blinking expectantly.

Max let Monty's words die away before beginning. It was abundantly clear than Dick did not want to be in this room, especially in these circumstances, and if he *had* to be, he wanted the whole business over and done with as speedily as possible and without too much controversy. Now Max was responsible for showing him that all of this was in fact important, and that he needed to focus.

'Thank you.' Max cleared his throat. 'First of all, I don't need to remind you that everything said in this room remains here. Confidentiality is vital. Now, the report. My wife, who has worked here for many years, gathered the information last month while in temporary charge of Grove House. She was shocked at what she found. Leaving aside administrative issues, some of the residents – two in particular – were clearly suffering from neglect. On page four is a photograph of a lady who has been kept in bed too long and not turned or washed frequently enough, so that her bedsores have become large, deep and infected. I do not think there can be any doubt that this is a case of neglect. Does anyone have anything to say on the matter?'

There were one or two expressions of remembered disgust in response to the picture, then Sandra spoke.

'Lil – that resident, I mean, was not in that state when I

was on the house. And I had the paperwork in order. It must have been Jean. I knew she wasn't up to it.'

'With respect,' Max replied, 'this kind of bedsore does not appear overnight. In one place the bone was visible.' He sensed Helen bristling near Sandra. He went on: 'The other resident in question was a slightly younger woman who, my wife recognised, was afflicted with a psychotic illness. There is a detailed account on page six of the kind of behaviour she displayed. It was clear to Mrs Greenwood that this resident had been confined to one room in the house for long periods, and had not been seen by a psychiatrist. She was ostracised by the other residents, who referred to her as "Nancy Nutter", and according to Catherine, a resident who knows everything that goes on in the house, she was deprived of food if she became aggressive. That is a denial of human rights. Has anyone got anything to say, or add, to this cata-logue?'

After a pause, Helen spoke up.

'Dr Greenwood is right to say that I was shocked at what I found on Grove. These two poor ladies really needed help. Lily is now in the ITU at Okebury Hospital with MRSA and Nancy is being treated in the psychiatric unit there.'

'What?' Sandra was indignant.

'Anybody else?'

'I find it hard to believe,' said Jim, standing up, scarcely able to contain himself, 'that this supposedly caring organi-sation, the nationally famous Squaremile Centre, which has its Investor in People award, can allow such dreadful things to happen to the vulnerable people living here. And it could all have been prevented! If the residents had had their My Life meetings, the care managers visiting from their home areas, not to mention the families, would have picked up on these problems before they got out of hand. Presumably Sandra didn't want anyone to see her residents though. But the finger should not only point to Sandra Wheatley. The Squaremile senior management must be held equally responsible for this shameful state of affairs. Incompetence, and I won't hesitate to use the word cruelty, has led to extreme suffering. There was no need for things to get this bad.'

As he sat down, he rapped his knuckles hard on the table and his face was dark with anger. Ms Olubi looked up from her note-taking. Max guessed Jim was not only thinking about Lily and Nancy at that moment.

'Have you anything to say, Mr Montgomery?' Max asked. Deprived of his chairmanship, Dick had been listening in silence, as had Jack Marshall.

'I have to accept responsibility,' Dick said quietly, deflated, 'on behalf of my staff, for these . . . serious occurrences. Of course things should have been handled better, and sooner.' One hand partly covered his mouth as he spoke, and his eyes darted from Sandra to Jack with ill-concealed disappointment. He grasped the side of the table again with the other hand; this time it was more as a support. He was scarcely audible now: 'This is a terrible state of affairs. It is not only neglect but abuse. I . . . '

' . . . So you will write to their families, then?' Jim was still agitated, 'And tell them that? You do realise that if this gets into the papers, Squaremile will be finished.'

'Yes.' Dick Montgomery seemed utterly defeated.

'I think . . . serious consideration needs to be given to the future of Squaremile's management team,' said Max. 'Can I suggest we have our coffee break now before moving on to Item 2 – shall we say half an hour? Thank you, ladies and gentlemen.'

'I'll take my drink in my office, Pat,' Dick Montgomery said to his secretary.

Neither Sandra nor Jack moved, so Max had to sidle past them to get to the door. The union rep followed them to the bar in the lounge. After only a few steps, they were still near enough to the boardroom to hear Jack shouting. Before Helen could speak, Max put his finger to his lips: 'Listen!' He whispered.

'I covered for you! I trusted you! Now my job's on the line. What do you propose to do about it?'

Then Helen and Max had to move away quickly, because

it seemed as though the door was about to be opened. Helen was pale. They went and bought coffee and sat in silence. She took some more painkillers. Meanwhile a beautiful day was in progress outside and ordinary life continued at Squaremile as if nothing significant was happening.

'I think a few heads will roll after this,' Max said softly.

Helen whispered: 'Oh, but Max! It was as if Dick hadn't even read the report. Did you see how his behaviour changed?'

'Yes, I thought the same thing.'

'I feel as if this is not really happening. We've been so wrapped up in it. But how am I supposed to go on working here now? That is, if . . . '

Jack appeared at the counter, red in the face and brusque with the waitress. He grabbed his cup and went smartly back in the direction of his own office, ignoring the Greenwoods. Ms Olubi took her drink back to the boardroom, with one for Sandra. Jim asked if he could sit with Max and Helen.

'Of course. Pleased you could make it, Jim,' said Helen, smiling, 'despite the circumstances.' Max went to buy Jim a coffee. As he returned, he heard Helen ask: 'Do you feel confident about Item 2?'

'After what we've seen so far this morning?' Jim was sensing victory. 'I should say so. It seems to be just a case of letting them hang themselves!'

Sandra didn't appear to have moved at all when they reassembled in the boardroom. She had obviously been discussing matters with the union rep; her papers were still spread out in front of her and she sat stony-faced as the others took their places. Pat was opening more windows. The boardroom really ought to be air-conditioned, Max thought, so that nothing could be heard from outside. Dick Montgomery was the last to return, still subdued.

'So, Item 2,' Max began, standing up. 'This concerns the treatment of the late Ms Victoria Gates while she was a care assistant at the Centre. I want it to be understood here that I am not in the habit of divulging anything about my patients, except perhaps to colleagues at the hospital. Even then, people remain anonymous unless and until someone needs to know about their case. On this occasion, however, I am obliged to reveal a certain amount of information in order to deal adequately with the issues in question, but only what is relevant. On these grounds I refuse, therefore, to discuss the nature and treatment of her illness.' He took a breath. 'To my mind, the Centre had a less than helpful attitude towards Ms Gates. It was known she had a problem when she was employed, yet – .'

'– We did not know the extent of that "problem" at the time,' Jack interrupted. 'You have to see this from our point of view. I mean, she took inordinate amounts of sick leave, which cost us money, and she could have become violent, or . . .'

'I think we have established that you have a duty of care towards your residents, don't you, Mr Marshall?' Suddenly all eyes were on Max, who realised he had raised his voice. He composed himself. 'In the same way, I have a duty of care towards my patients. And as I said in answer to the questions you sent me when she was working here, there was no likelihood of violent or aggressive behaviour. I'm assuming you did see those answers, that they were forwarded from Personnel?'

Dick nodded.

'Nobody was in danger. Ms Gates was known as a hard-working member of the staff team on Forest House. Brendan Donnelly, her first boss, valued the skills she could offer: she was a trained teacher looking for a new career. She didn't know if or when she would be ill, but every time she was at her most vulnerable, when she had been in hospital, when she needed support, how did Squaremile respond? By talking to her and trying to help? No! By subjecting her to a disciplinary hearing each time and issuing warnings, by punishing her for something she could not help. That is unfair!'

Dick Montgomery spoke at last. 'Er, are you unwell, Dr Greenwood? You seem a little unsteady on your feet, that's all. Shouldn't you be taking some sort of medication for the old ticker? We wouldn't want *you* off sick again, would we?'

Sandra smirked.

'No sir. It's just hot in here', replied Max.

He had stopped Max in full flow, deliberately, as if he could not completely relinquish control. After another pause, Dick grimaced, suggesting that a compromise was coming:

'In connection with those hearings, I do agree that the term "disciplinary" was inappropriate, unfortunate even, and I said as much at the time, but we had to do *something*.' He leant forward in a travesty of confiding in Max. 'As much as anything, you understand, we had to let other junior staff be shown that lengthy absences would not be tolerated, you know.' He finished with an assertive nod and frown.

'In other words, Vee was used as an example?' Max replied. 'And do you think that she could – to use your word – *tolerate* being ill? Have you the slightest notion of what it's like to have your world ripped apart by an illness like this?'

Dick studied Max for a moment. 'I admit, I have no personal experience of mental illness, but you are a psychiatrist, so . . . '

'Yes, and in my professional judgement, the Centre exacerbated her condition. She did not *choose* to be ill, or do it to annoy others, or for attention. Life was made even more difficult for her by being here. In my view, residents and staff should be treated with the same degree of respect.'

Dick folded his hands together in front of him on the table.

'So in your opinion, a couple of hearings and warnings drove her to suicide, Mr Chairman. Is that what you expect us to believe?' The Chief Executive's confidence seemed to have returned; he was adopting his dismissive stance once more, complete with the glasses act. Max continued.

'Oh no. It was much *more* than that. Ms Gates was eventually promoted, then moved, after the fire on Alder, to Grove House, run at the time by Ms Wheatley. I believe that, in the first instance, Sandra was jealous of Vee's qualifications, and saw her as a threat.'

Sandra was staring at Max. Then she flung herself back in her seat, shaking her head and smiling incredulously. 'You *are* joking! I can't believe I'm hearing this! You've got a bloody nerve!'

'That's how it appeared, from what Ms Gates told me.'

'And you'd believe the word of a . . . a . . . ' Sandra's eyes darted round the group.

'A what, Ms Wheatley?' Max collected his thoughts again, trying to concentrate and ignore the feeling in his chest. There was no reply. 'Whether it's true or not, you soon found her Achilles heel. You gave her a hard time, I know that. I can only conclude that you allowed your personal feelings to get in the way of a professional, working relationship of the kind Ms Gates enjoyed on her first house. Vee's illness became your preoccupation. You gave her no credit for doing a good job when she was well. Everybody knew she worked hard – relied on it, in fact. I have read what Vee wrote about you.' Max was building to a climax. 'If you hadn't bullied her, we might not have needed this meeting because she might still have been alive.' With that he sat down.

'How dare you say such a thing! Flinging wild accusations at me! And don't you think the way she died goes to prove she wasn't up to it?' Sandra lost her cool, as he'd hoped she would. Everyone in the room was aware of the tension. Sandra looked at Ms Olubi, shook her head in mock despair and shrugged as if she didn't have any idea what Max meant; but her reaction had already shown the opposite. Ms Olubi stared at her, then went on writing notes.

'Fascinating, I'm sure, Dr Greenwood,' said Dick Montgomery, with a cough. 'But there's something missing in all this: you have given us no *evidence* whatsoever for the claims you make regarding Ms Gates. This is all hearsay, empty allegations.' And – he raised his hand to prevent comment, 'I think our chairman is too involved with the case.'

'We can't change the chairman half way through the meeting!' Helen exclaimed in her Scots accent.

'Unless that chairman is ill.' Dick threw Max a glance, eyebrows raised.

Jim stepped in: 'Look, since when did anyone have to prove their innocence, eh? What happened to "innocent until proven guilty"?' He was becoming more and more frustrated. 'What I'm trying to say is, what evidence can *you* produce, Sandra, to prove Vee was doing anything wrong? No resident was injured or died as a result of her actions, did they?'

'What about June and Catherine in the Alder House fire?' Sandra was desperate.

'But Vee didn't *start* the fire, did she? And where were you when she was getting people out to safety, eh?' Jim glared at her.

The intensity of the meeting was taking its toll. At the same time, Max was anxious not to let anyone else take over, or for things to get out of hand.

'Presumably you thought you were doing the right thing, Ms Wheatley,' he continued. 'Treating Vee as you did. For yourself, perhaps, your own advancement. Now, Mr Montgomery, you say you want evidence. My wife and I were aware that you would, so Helen interviewed the junior staff who knew Sandra in Birch and Grove.'

'So you got your wife to do the dirty work?'

'I suppose you could say that, but she is on the spot. She recorded the interviews, two of which I propose to play to you now. But before we come to that, I would like to suggest that we take our lunch break now. This morning's business has taken longer than expected. Shall we reconvene at two o'clock?'

As he stood up, Dick Montgomery said, 'I've no doubt a good many of your patients would like you to be their champion, Dr Greenwood. Are you planning any more sorties into other organisations, I wonder? Flying the flag of justice? With a flick of his eyebrows, he added, 'I wasn't aware that a psychiatrist's job was to treat the whole world, especially when he is unwell himself.'

28

The Boardroom (2)

'This is not normal practice,' said Ms Olubi, sitting down and nodding her head in the direction of the tape recorder. 'There had better be a good reason for it.'

Helen replied, 'I think the recordings allow an insight into everyday life on a house and into Sandra's behaviour, two things which we would probably not be able to convey to the meeting in any other way.' She moved to the other end of the table, opposite Jim, and set up the cassette player.

Max remembered their practice run at home the night before. 'Perhaps, Mrs Greenwood, you would be kind enough to talk us through them.'

'Thank you, er, Mr Chairman. In the office at Grove, I interviewed several staff who had worked with Sandra in Alder, Grove and Birch, with their knowledge and consent. Of these recordings, some had too much background noise or were interrupted beyond saving, and one was too faint to be of any use. The two remaining are fairly self-explanatory.'

She reached into her bag for the tapes. After some frantic rummaging, she looked up in horror. 'They're not here! I put them ready in this bag last night! With the player!' She stared at Max. 'You didn't take them out for any reason, did you?'

'No. Didn't touch them.'

'Please excuse me, everybody, but I need a word with my husband outside.' She closed the door quietly and they stood in the corridor. 'I *know* I put them in there! Last night!' Helen's desperation showed once again in her Scots accent.

'Just stop and think for a minute. Did you leave the bag unattended at all this morning, when you were on the house?'

'Oh . . . yes . . . it's coming back to me. I had to leave the office to go and help somebody.'

'Who else was around?'

'The usual staff.' They looked at each other intently. 'But why?' asked Helen.

'Hey, a motive isn't hard to find, is it?' Max opened the boardroom door. Helen slipped in as he spoke: 'We are going to have to adjourn while we try to find the tapes. It would not be easy to proceed without them.'

Everybody groaned and started to move; Max noticed the crooked smile on Sandra's face.

'We'd better have a re-start time, then,' said Dick. 'We'll give you until three o'clock. Back here then, ladies and gents.'

The room emptied quickly, leaving the two of them.

'Before we do anything else,' Helen muttered, 'I must get some more painkillers. I feel terrible.'

'Poor darling!'

They walked back to Grove House together. Nat was at the window. He'd never been inside, and this was Helen's territory, so he let her lead the way. It was very quiet as most of the residents were at Activities, Helen explained. Nat was standing by the door now, and they followed her into the office without a word.

'Lookin' for these?' she asked, swinging round and holding up the tapes. She wore an expression which said, "Go on, challenge me!" Helen reached out for the tapes but Nat jerked her arm away.

'Oh no! Did you really fink we woz gunna let you tape us, then use it against Sandra? She knew. Oh yeah – we worked it out!'

'Nat, give me the tapes, please.' Helen was trying to stay calm.

'Are they *really* important then?' Nat giggled. 'Hey, you're that shrink, innit?'

'I am a psychiatrist, yes.'

'Did ya know Vee?' Nat was still laughing because of her perceived power over them.

'Yes.'

'Ha, ha!' She could hardly contain herself. 'I s'pose Helen here's another one of your patients then. Go round lookin' for nutters, collectin' 'em, do ya?' Neither of them could answer. 'Well?' She was still holding the tapes in the air.

They didn't respond, until finally Helen said: 'I'll forget what you just said if you let me have the tapes.'

'Wassit worth? Go on!'

'If you give them back, I shan't say anything about your behaviour – Oh! I'm sorry, Liz, but nobody else is allowed in the office at the moment!' The girl walked away and Helen shut the door and faced Nat. 'You won't be disciplined.'

'Pha! Thass no good. I wuz gunna leave this dump soon anyway. I dunt give a *monkey's* about discipline!'

The three of them stood motionless.

'I know what,' said Nat, 'I get to come to the big fat boss meetin' you're 'avin."

'But you ca – ' Helen began, but Max interrupted her. '– If you give us the tapes, you can sit in.'

Silently, with false reluctance, Nat handed over the cassettes, having slipped them quickly into a carrier bag. A stupid grin spread across her face.

It was five past three. Everyone was back in the boardroom except Sandra. Once again, Dick looked at his watch. Max put his briefcase next to Helen's bag. Jack coughed. Ms Olubi found the right page in her notes, pulled her chair in and fiddled with her earrings. Nat came in, walked casually round behind the Chief Executive and sat next to Max.

'Does anyone know where Sandra is?' Max began. Some said "no" while others shook their heads.

'We have managed to find the tapes,' Helen said, as she plugged in the cassette player for a second time.

'Excuse me,' said Dick, 'but what is this junior member of staff doing in here?'

Helen stayed calm. 'I said she could join us to get experience of meetings.'

'But the matters we are discussing are of a confidential nature!'

'Sir, I think we can rely on Ms Cooper's discretion.' Helen looked hard at Nat, then went on: 'Now, as I said earlier, only two of the recordings I made were any good and – oh, no!' Helen shrieked in dismay.

'What's wrong now, Mrs Greenwood?' Dick's impatience came partly from having missed his lunch engagement.

'They've been *cut!*' Helen noticed as soon as she took the cassettes from their cases. She stood up abruptly, turned on Nat, who was laughing, and shouted: '*Get out!* Get out of this room! You haven't heard the last of this!'

Nat obeyed, still grinning. Jim took one of the cassettes and passed it round. There were murmurs of disbelief.

'Whatever's going on?' asked Dick.

'Sir, we've been sabotaged. But all is not lost,' Max replied. 'I have copies of the transcripts I made in case of power failure, or something unexpected like this. They don't have the same impact, but it's probably for the best in the end so that we don't recognise the voices.'

'Wouldn't they have been better in your report booklet?' Dick pointed out.

'Possibly. But this is particularly sensitive material. I'll have the copies back afterwards please.'

There was still no sign of Sandra, however. Everyone started to read the transcripts which Max passed round, before all sight of their purpose was lost.

FIRST INTERVIEW

HELEN: How long have you worked here, at Squaremile?

ANON 1: 'Bout five years. [Max remembered that this was Liz.]

HELEN: So you came here straight from school?

ANON 1: Yeah. I started on Birch, before Bill, ven came here, ven got promoted.

HELEN: Are you happy here?

ANON 1: Pretty much. 'Sonly a job though, innit? Not worth gettin' stressed about.

Pause

HELEN: Can I ask you . . . about Vee. Did you get on with her?

ANON 1: Yeah, but I di'n't fink she was right in vis job.

HELEN: What do you mean?

ANON 1: Well, she 'ad degrees an' that. Dunno why she came here.

HELEN: You're saying she was overqualified.

ANON 1: Yeah, pretty much, yeah. Dunno what she was doin' 'ere. I know it got to some people. Vee sometimes 'ad a good idea, y'know, but because it was *'er* that thought of it . . . People got jealous, y'see.

HELEN: I see. (Thinks for a moment.) Can I ask you now what you thought of Sandra, as a manager, I mean?

ANON 1: She was OK, I s'pose. More laid back than Jenny used to be in Birch, before Bill, y'know, but she – Sandra I mean – was dead keen to keep the place clean more than anythin' else, for visitors an' that.

HELEN: Did she get on with the residents?

ANON 1: Yeah, but we 'ad to do all the work wiv them. Still, she was the manager, so I s'pose she could do what she liked.

HELEN: Hmm. Did Sandra get on with Vee?

ANON 1: Oh, no, not really. Dunno why, 'cos Vee worked as 'ard as the rest of us.

HELEN: Vee worked hard, did she?

ANON 1: Oh, yeah! Always on da go. 'Cept when she was ill o' course.

HELEN: Was Sandra different in any way when Vee was there and when she wasn't?

ANON 1: Erm, let's fink. I fink she was a bit 'appier wiv Vee not around, but she . . .

(The telephone rings.)

HELEN: Hello? Yes. Is it urgent? Only I'm in a meeting right now. OK. Bye. Sorry, you were saying?

ANON 1: Erm, I don't fink Sandra wanted Vee around. When Vee come back, it was like Sandra dint care. She gave 'er grief an' that. Know wha' I mean?

HELEN: What kind of grief?

ANON 1: Oh, I dunno. Always pickin' up on fings, criticisin' an' givin' 'er nasty jobs like cleanin' a blocked toilet or somebody's . . . Hey, you're not goin' to report me for this, are you? 'Cos I don't fink it's right to take sides a' work. I wan' you to know that. It's just a job, like I said.

HELEN: Don't worry.

ANON 1: There's sumfin' else. Sandra told us that Vee was goin' to 'ave to go. We 'ad to give 'er – Sandra I mean – a piece of paper every week for free weeks sayin' what Vee 'ad done wrong. There 'ad to be at least free fings on da paper each time, so I fink some people made stuff up, just so Sandra wunt get annoyed.

(End.)

The silence of the boardroom gradually gave way to coughs and whispered conversations as people finished reading.

'Perhaps we can have comments when you've all read the second interview,' Max said. He knew that this was Nat. 'If anything, it illustrates the problem better.'

SECOND INTERVIEW

HELEN: Do you like this job?

ANON 2: 'S alright. When people don't nag. (Sounds of chewing.)

HELEN: OK. I want to ask you a few questions. Any information you give won't be used against you. I won't nag on this. If you don't want to answer a question, that's fine, but it would be helpful if you do. I have seen your helpful side. I will not tell anyone who said what in any case.

ANON 2: Right, go on, then. (Still sounding a little defensive.)

HELEN: How long have you known Sandra?

ANON 2: About . . . three years.

HELEN: Do you like her? Do you think she is a good manager?

ANON 2: Yes. She's been good to me, given me chances, basic'ly. Shown me the ropes an' stuff.

HELEN: So you were sorry when she got promoted off the house.

ANON 2: Yep. Jean was nice, but a bit soft. Then there was you.

HELEN: Did you get on with Vee too?

ANON 2: Ah, she was off 'er 'ead that one.

HELEN: So you didn't get on with her.

ANON 2: I don't mix with that sort. Sandra reckoned she should've stayed in the funny farm for good. You never knew what she might do next, basic'ly.

(Anon 2 giggles.) [Max remembered realising that Helen seemed to have found a topic on which Nat had strong views.]

HELEN: What makes you say that?

ANON 2: Every so often she'd 'ave a funny turn an' go off sick. I reckon she was lazy, as well as nuts. That sort shouldn't be in work, because they make it harder for the rest of us in the end. Sandra said Vee couldn't do anything right, wha'ever she did. People like 'er should be put away and forgotten, basic'ly, so the rest of us can get on with our lives, the useless ... (Anon 2 cannot think of a strong enough insult beyond swearing. She coughs instead.) I know Sandra felt the same, and I trusted her. We used to have a laugh!

(Audible amusement.)

HELEN [sounding rather annoyed, as Max recalled]: What about the fire? Didn't she get everyone out on her own?

ANON 2: She was only doin' her job. Anyone else would've done the same. And for all we knew, she could've started it 'erself! Yeah, she could've 'eard a voice tellin' er to start a fire! Well, we don't know what goes on in their 'eads, do we? That sort like a bit of attention, too.

HELEN [Max could picture her expression as he read]: But the fact remains, she rescued those residents. She wasn't behaving oddly then, was she?

ANON 2: You on Vee's side?

HELEN: I don't think there are any "sides" in this.

(End.)

Sandra finally put in an appearance and took her place next to Ms Olubi. 'I'm sorry. I was needed elsewhere,' she said, in response to a questioning look from Dick Montgomery.

'Right. I suggest you read these two interviews, Ms Wheatley,' he said crisply, while the rest of us take a short break. Ten minutes, then.'

They left Sandra with Ms Olubi. Jim, Helen and Max sat with their coffee in the dismal staff lounge, in silence. Jack had vanished, but when he returned with Dick, they all filed back into the boardroom once again.

'This has got to have been concocted by you!' The words burst from Sandra as she stood up suddenly, knocking her chair over, shaking the papers she held out in front of her, glaring at Max. 'Who do you think you are, playing God?' She turned and looked from Jack Marshall to Dick Montgomery. 'It's not fair! You *asked* me to get rid of her! I was doing what *you* wanted!' She was shouting, incensed, still clutching the sheets of paper. 'You said it was the only way forward, the only thing to do, for the good of Squaremile! You said you would back me and see me right!'

'You didn't have to accept,' Dick pointed out coldly. 'Or go to such apparent lengths.' He looked at Jack, who seemed anxious.

Helen could hardly contain herself. 'And you didn't have to treat her so badly! Having interviewed your staff, I heard things which made me think you actually *enjoyed* making Vee's life a misery! It didn't take you much effort to do what they asked. And you have the audacity, now, to say this isn't fair on *you!* And while I'm at it, I suppose we all know why you never had a Professional Conduct Review, don't we?' She glared at Jack. 'And all those hearings *Vee* had to go to – they were for the wrong person!' Helen was trembling. She knocked over her glass and Max made to help her, but she found a tissue before the water got to the report.

Jim was tight-lipped, scowling in silence. Janice Olubi

appeared utterly amazed, looking from one person to another with her mouth half open.

Sandra righted her chair and sat down, trying to compose herself. 'I did what I thought was right,' she said in a low voice. 'I don't think that kind of person should be in a job like this, or any other job, for that matter.'

'What kind of person is that, then, exactly?' Jim spoke with controlled anger.

Sandra just stared at him. The room was very warm. Max took off his jacket.

Helen spoke to Jack Marshall: 'There's one other thing I'd like to clear up, while I have the opportunity. After Sandra had collected "evidence", mainly false, from her minions, you had the meeting where Vee was accused of all kinds of malpractice, yes?'

Jack could not help looking sheepish after the earlier attack.

'I remember. And we had Dr Greenwood's answers in support of Vee around the same time.'

'Well,' she went on, 'were you aware that Vee had not *seen* the list of allegations before the meeting? Nor did she realise she was being watched on the house and that notes were being made in preparation for it. That's what Anon 1 was referring to. The first Vee knew of the whole business was when she was called in to face the firing squad. She didn't even have notice of the meeting itself!'

Jack thought for a moment. 'I was not aware of that, no.' He stared at Sandra and spoke with quiet anger, his voice deep: 'You told me that she knew what was going on, that she'd seen the list and she was willing to come. Are there any other . . . irregularities we should know about, while you've got the chance?'

Sandra did not respond.

Max stood up. 'At that meeting, planned weeks in advance, nobody was prepared to believe Vee. The so-called evidence was weighted against her: it was a prearranged defeat.' He took a sip of water. 'Ladies and gentlemen, I think we now have a better picture of how things have been running. I also think we know what has to be done. What is your opinion, Ms Olubi?'

He sat down; he was perspiring and he tried to breathe deeply out of fear for his heart. Helen pulled her chair over to join him. The pain in her head bloomed like an atomic mushroom cloud; at the same time she was aware of the danger for her husband. She listened with her eyes closed behind one hand for a moment, holding Max's hand under the table with the other. She thought she was going to pass out.

'I would expect immediate resignations from the staff concerned,' Ms Olubi replied. 'Mr Montgomery will have to attend a separate hearing with the trustees and someone from the Charity Commission, but – .'

'– As I said in reply to Item 1,' Dick broke in, 'I accept full responsibility. Item 2 has provided further evidence that more care needs to be exercised in the appointment of staff.'

Max looked at Dick in disbelief. 'If you mean in terms of not employing someone with a mental health problem,' he said, 'how can you possibly know in advance who will develop one?'

'What makes you think I am referring to Ms Gates?'

At that point, Sandra left the room, angry, with a dismissive glance at Ms Olubi. There was a long pause. It seemed that everybody felt there was something else which needed to be said, but nobody could articulate it.

'Any other business?'

> «*Si 'Eternel existe,*
> *en fin de compte*
> *Il voit qu'*
> *je me conduis*
> *guère plus mal*
> *Que si j'avais la foi.*»
> GEORGES BRASSENS

29
Anxiety

Jim went back with Max and Helen that night. In spite of their exhaustion, everyone had to eat. Then they talked until late.

'I am so grateful to you both for letting me witness the apocalypse! But I'm sorry you're not well, Helen. Good luck for tomorrow. Let me know if there's anything you need.'

Max knew the reason why Helen had wanted to talk so late that night. She was trying to avoid thinking about today. As if to prove it, now that they were on their way to Okebury, she picked up the topic of Squaremile again, despite being weary and in need of quiet. She spoke with her eyes closed, as if by talking, by skating lightly over the surface of her emotions, she could simultaneously distract herself and prepare for what was about to happen. But they did not need to discuss any of this because each knew what the other was thinking.

'You were a brilliant chairman. I know I've said it before, but . . . And you know when Monty said I'd done your dirty work for you, well, I couldn't help thinking how that applied to Sandra as well. You were right when you said she was acting for them, but they gave her too much freedom. They assumed she was good at her job and they didn't know what she was really – .'

'– Helen, Helen!' He had to stop her, gently, with a sigh, because her anxiety was beginning to affect him. They pulled into the hospital car park.

'Sorry, Max. I do go on a bit sometimes, don't I? You know me.'

'Yes, darling.' They found the MRI department easily. 'Good luck. I'll be waiting for you.'

The metallic heartbeat of the scanner made her apprehensive as she was shown into the white room with the giant, humming machine. Assistants came and went.

'Have you brought your earplugs?' someone asked her. 'Only it can get very loud in there. And forgive me if I'm repeating myself, but I have to ask if you have any metallic objects in or on your body?'

She had given her watch and bag to Max. She took off her shoes and lay on the bed. They adjusted her position. Before long she was gliding into the narrow tunnel and she experienced a momentary claustrophobia, which she had to fight rationally. She found it helped if she closed her eyes and imagined she was lying in a field with open sky above her, rather in than a tube whose wall was only two or three inches from her nose.

'Don't move now. Stay absolutely still,' came a voice over the microphone.

Now the giant's heartbeat stepped up to a bang, bang, bang, then a bidoon, bidoon, bidoon, followed by a series of other loud sequences, sometimes scratchy, not always in bass. These unpredictable sounds became her whole existence for a long period; she had been told it could take up to an hour and a half. The feeling of powerlessness washed away all other thoughts, which could not co-exist with the demands on her ears. She felt as though she had turned into a subterranean rock at the mercy of erosion. Eventually, the rhythmic sounds reduced in intensity. She felt cold. The microphone crackled: 'All done now, Mrs Greenwood.'

The bed moved silently out of the tunnel and the heartbeat faded back to a muffled hum-thump, with a top note that sounded like a distant, automated forge.

'You'll get the results within a week,' said one of the assistants. 'If you'd like to make an appointment with your GP.'

'The news is mixed,' said Dr Conway.

'Please tell us, doctor,' Max had come in with her and held her hand while the doctor spoke.

'You have a brain tumour, Mrs Greenwood.'

She coughed. 'I . . . I had a feeling it might be that.' She pinched the bridge of her nose, trying to stop the welling up of emotion and at the same time absorb the information which was now horribly real, no longer an abstraction.

'But you said the news was mixed,' said Max.'What do you mean?'

'Well, there is some good news.' Dr Conway sat back and rested his elbows on the arms of his chair. 'Firstly, there do not appear to be any tumours elsewhere in your body; secondly the growth is not too large. It's large enough to cause problems, yes, but . . . And thirdly, its location is such that removal should not be too difficult.' He smiled professionally. 'Do you have any questions?'

Helen screwed up her courage. 'Well, yes actually. Will there be any . . . after effects? I mean, will there be any . . . damage?'

'It's unlikely as we seem to have caught it in time.'

'Is it cancerous?'

'Most tumours like this are benign, but there is a possibility, yes. It looks as if it might be what they call "encapsulated", in other words kept separate from other brain tissues. But they will have to do a biopsy to be able to tell anything else for sure.'

'Will I have the kind of surgery where I'm awake and can talk to you?'

'Not on this occasion, no.'

'One more thing: how long will it be before I can have the operation? You see, my daughter's graduation is coming up soon.'

'And we've got a holiday booked for August, too,' added Max, squeezing Helen's hand. She smiled at him. He felt he needed to give Helen something.

'I should think we're talking . . . two weeks' time? I'll arrange for you to have your pre-op assessment next week. Wednesday suit you?'

'Fine. So we can carry on with our plans then?'

'I don't see why not. You can spend your holiday relaxing and convalescing. Where are you going?'

'Oh, I can't say at the moment,' said Max. 'I'm not giving *everything* away. It was meant to be a surprise.'

'Well, I'll see you when you've had the biopsy. And Helen, don't forget that support is available.'

Max pushes open the door to the lecture theatre and tries to switch on the lights. Only one will come on: his spotlight on the platform. He becomes aware that the students are sitting there in the dark, waiting patiently.

"We thought you weren't coming back again, Dr Greenwood," says one voice. Strangely, however, the atmosphere doesn't feel at all hostile. Max steps into the circle of light. This time, the faces are not illuminated when they speak.

"I needed to think," he replies, placing one hand on each side of the lectern.

"What did you need to think about?" This is a different voice.

"Does anyone believe in God?"

Nobody speaks; now he might as well be addressing an empty room.

"Does anyone believe in death?"

"Sir." It is a girl's voice. "What do you mean by believe? It's just something that happens, a natural conclusion."

"What I mean is, is death the end?"

"Why are you asking us these questions?" says another, deeper voice, more curious than anything else. "Do you think we have prepared for this?"

Max remembered Bella saying once that Vee didn't believe in God. At least, not the kind of God who would allow evil and suffering to flourish in the world as they have always done. Religious faith was something he'd practically ignored, claiming the typically British "CofE" label when necessary on forms, as if to put him in a kind of safe place, just in case people were right all along. But he knew he was avoiding the issue, hedging his bets. Now seemed as good a time as any to examine his beliefs once and for all.

He did not need to look far; he had to agree with Vee. Devastation, degradation, illness and cruelty would not be allowed to happen on such a scale if God loved the world, and as for the "cop out" that He gave us free will, it could surely have been curtailed in some way by a being with such power, omniscience and supposed benevolence. Max was certainly not going to expound some theory about mankind, but he did believe humans were meant to help each other, and other creatures, especially if there was no higher power. Oh, he knew this to be a centuries-old, well-worn path, but he felt he had to focus on these things at this point in his life. He could not avoid thinking about the possibility of Helen's death, or incapacity.

The idea was sobering. If he carried his argument through, there was nothing afterwards. And if he believed that, why couldn't he accept that the world would just go on as if she hadn't happened? That must be the ultimate cruelty. We would all like to believe that something of us remains, that we have some personal impact, or that our souls watch over our loved ones. But how will we know if there is a resurrection until it's too late? He also had to ask himself if he was becoming depressed, with all this introspection on mortality. Perhaps, but he wanted to put it down to apprehension. In fact it was more likely to be terror.

Max drove Helen to her preoperative assessment that Wednesday. Everything was fine: blood pressure, weight, ECG reading and blood test. She told the doctor of the operations she'd had up to now: appendectomy aged fifteen, then the resetting of a compound fracture of her lower leg when she was a student and so on. The detailed examination and conversation lasted about two hours and she emerged exhausted. She slept part of the way home in the car. She had the biopsy to face the next day.

While he thought Helen was still asleep, driving on

through the countryside, Max felt that Vee was there with him again; this time it was not jealousy that emanated from her but a feeling of peace. He couldn't explain why Vee came to him, or how he knew she was there.

He recalled what she'd written, about her attitude to mental illness while she was young, how it had changed and then how she was derided by people who still held the same views she had been forced to abandon. Perhaps they too, he and Helen, were being punished for assuming they would never become ill. But by whom? An angry, vengeful God? He was back in the theological debate. But whatever people believed, health is a more delicate thing than most imagine, especially when viewed by the young.

His thoughts turned to another patient. He would call her Miss X. She was mildly depressed and anxious and looking for stability. Somehow she obtained his home phone number and called several times. Despite being in her twenties, she obviously had a crush on him, and kept repeating that she "needed" him. All Max could do was reassure her, change his number and go ex-directory. That was years ago. Everybody in his line of work *had* to be ex-directory these days. More to the point, was he *needed* now? He knew he needed Helen, but he was completely retired now, so he wasn't needed by anyone at work. He was, however, facing challenges over which he had limited control, for himself and his dear Helen. *She* needed him; his anxiety centred on whether he was strong enough to support her.

'Oh, you're awake,' said Max, turning into their road. 'Here we are, darling. You go up and I'll bring you a cup of tea.'

It was only five o'clock but it felt like midnight. She didn't remember anything until she woke up in the early hours needing some painkillers, still fully dressed apart from her shoes, and lying on top of the bed. Max was in bed beside her, sound asleep. In the dim light, she noticed how his relaxed face was beginning to show his age.

On the day of the operation, he helped her get dressed and

into the car; she didn't care that she couldn't have breakfast. The next thing she knew, she was on a hospital trolley,
with corridor lights flashing, passing overhead. It was very
quiet to begin with in the theatre. Dr Conway had told her
what the biopsy had revealed: it was malignant. It had to
come out. A gowned figure looked at her as if from a great
height.

'Hello, Helen. I'm Mr McDonald. I'll be performing your
operation. You'll be fine.'

'Oh, a fellow Scot!' She remembered Vee's description of
anaesthesia. The oxygen mask, the cold trickle making her
aware of her vein . . .

She wondered what the flashing lights were overhead.
Then she realised that it was all over and she was being taken
along the corridor again. She closed her eyes. She seemed to
be wearing a hat . . . The trolley rumbled as it turned a corner
into a small ward. Shoes squeaked on the floor. She was
moved on to the cold sheets of a bed and attached to moni-
tors. The nurse busied herself with the equipment. Helen
tried to speak but could not utter a sound to begin with. The
hat throbbed when she coughed. Then:

'Has it gone, Mum?' Her voice sounded strange and she
had a sore throat.

'Has wha . . . Oh!' said the young Asian nurse. 'Yes, it's
gone. Now get some rest, Mrs Greenwood, and I'll be back
in a little while.' Helen realised that her mother wasn't there.
Then gradually, as her thoughts began to clear even more,
she recalled the recent events at Squaremile.

'Hello, my brave, beautiful lady.' Max was sitting by the
bed now and he spoke softly. 'How are you feeling?'

She reached out and looked at his watch. Several hours
had passed unnoticed! She croaked: 'OK I think. Got a
terrible headache, but it's different. What does my hat look
like?'

Max laughed lightly. 'Want some water?' He poured half
a cup from the plastic jug. 'Nurse, I think my wife needs
some pain relief please.'

The nurse spoke quietly. 'She can use the PCA, Mr

Greenwood.' She came over to them from another patient who was asleep. 'I'll show you what to do. See this? You just press that and it delivers some morphine.'

'Oh, yes. Thank you.' Max had forgotten about PCAs, he said. Helen pressed the button and felt suddenly lighter and more hopeful. She smiled at Max. 'Have you told the girls?'

'Yes, my love. They were quite worried, but I told them they couldn't visit until I had made sure that you were up to it.'

'I feel fine! How long am I meant to stay here?' She felt her bandage. Max could tell that she was far from fine.

'Until they're satisfied you can manage and you've healed a bit. They'll have to do some tests, but Mr Mc Donald reckons you should make a full recovery. I spoke to him while you were asleep, but he'll come and talk to you tomorrow, I expect. You'll be a bit bruised.' He stroked her hand. 'I've missed you, Helen. We've all been praying for you.'

'Praying?'

'Well, not exactly, but you know what I mean. Hoping strongly, willing everything to be alright.' He smiled. 'But I've got a confession to make – or is *that* the wrong word to use?!'

Helen groaned. 'Enough already. Well? What have, or haven't, you done?'

'I told Grace and Anna about the tumour the night after we'd been told. I couldn't really leave it til now, could I? It would have been too much all at once.'

'It's OK, Max.' She must have drifted off to sleep again to Max's voice and the sounds of the ward, because when she next opened her eyes, Grace and Anna were sitting by the bed with their father. Max had given the girls the OK. They had spent the night in a local hotel, at his expense. Their faces lit up when they saw that Helen knew them.

'Hello, Mum,' said Anna. 'You know I'm going to be staying with Dad for a few days?'

Not to be left out, Grace took her mother's hand. 'Hey! And you'd better be coming to my graduation!'

'Wouldn't miss it for the world, sweetheart! I want to know when I'm getting out of here!'

'Helen,' said Max, trying to calm her. 'There's someone else here who'd like to see you. Come on girls, let's leave them to it.'

Helen lay back on a sun lounger in shorts and the vest Anna had bought her for her birthday. As Max put a glass of orange juice on the table beside her, the paperback she had been reading slipped to the floor.

'I could get used to this, Max! Thank you darling. Have you got the sun cream?' They had a villa on the Côte d'Azur for three weeks. Max sat on the other lounger, feeling very lazy, but he didn't see why he should feel guilty. He had managed to finish writing up the details of the Squaremile showdown before they left. These notes, intended originally to help him with regard to Vee's inquest, had almost developed into his own novel. He would let Helen read them sometime.

He felt warm and comfortable – and relieved: Helen's follow-up scan had shown the absence of cancer. When the bandages came off, she had a shaved area on the left side. Helen had joked that they were trying to match his hairstyle. She said she was just relieved to be rid of the thing, with all its unpleasant effects, and that she only had a grain-sized headache now, as opposed to a football.

Helen had been so happy she'd cried when her mum came to see her on the ward. It was quite a journey from Edinburgh for an elderly lady, but she had been worried when Max got in touch. While her mother was stroking Helen's face, Max had noticed the same expression of warmth in her eyes as he had seen many times in Helen's. It was one of the special things which had first attracted him to her. He did not stand around after that to hear what was said, but his mother-in-law stayed with Max and Anna for a few days, until after Helen was allowed home.

All they could hear now were the relentless cicadas. Then

Helen's mobile rang. She felt in her bag. 'Damn! I meant to switch that thing off and leave the world behind . . . Hello, Anna! What's the matter?'

Almost immediately, Helen stood up and walked over to the other end of the verandah, and was looking out to sea with her back to Max. As the conversation progressed, he could tell the news was not good. The tone of her voice suggested both surprise and anxiety, and his curiosity was mounting. She came back towards him. 'I'll tell your dad, yes. He's fine, taking it easy for once. Have you heard from Grace, by the way? Oh, that's good. We did enjoy her special day. I know, shame there were only two tickets. But it'll be your turn soon! Right. Good. Thanks Anna. Bye.'

She closed the phone. 'Well, Grace is OK, anyway. She deserves a holiday after all her hard work. She arrived safely in Lausanne last night, with Dan. She's wanted to go back to Switzerland for ages – .'

'– Yes, yes, I know, but come on! What was the rest of it about?'

Helen sighed and sat down. 'It seems we can't get away from the Centre, even in the south of France! Squaremile has made the national news, Max. Dick Montgomery's body was found in his office and, in the euphemistic phrase they use, the police are "not looking for anyone else". He hanged himself, Max.' She picked up her glass and took a mouthful. 'And there's more. Not only is Sandra out of a job, she's been arrested! Someone went to the press with a story of neglected residents and "irregularities" in the way staff were treated at Squaremile.'

Max whispered, '*Yes!*' in triumph, and then asked, 'Do we know who told the papers?'

'You and I both have our suspicions on that one, but we may never know for sure. But it looks as if I'll have to find another job when we get back, doesn't it?'

'It does.'

'So much for going back part-time in Sycamore. It's a shame, because I'm only ten years off retirement. Perhaps you'll have ageism to combat next!'

'Oh, no, no, I've fought all the battles I intend to, thank you very much. I want a quiet life now.'

'Are you saying,' said Helen in mock indignation, 'that you wouldn't take up the cudgels on my behalf?'

'Only if absolutely necessary – and if you didn't give me any peace!'

They laughed and Helen tried to tickle his chest, where the little curl of grey hair was, right in the middle. They stood up and walked arm in arm across the wooden boards to the rail. Helen looked glamorous in her sunglasses as they counted the distant boats under a cloudless sky.

'I wonder what Jim's made of the headlines,' she said.

'I can't believe it. And just think, it's nearly a whole year since his sister died.'

Max took a mouthful of his drink. 'Poor Monty, though, eh? I feel sorry for him in spite of what he represented.'

'Yes, I heard his wife died back in November, so the trouble at work must've been the last straw.

'Sounds like it. But to psychoanalyse Monty would have been interesting. I don't think he knew half of what was going on at the Centre, but he obviously believed in it. The ship that could never sink.'

They went back to the loungers.

'Hey, let's forget about home now. This holiday is my present to you, so we'll do whatever you want, bearing in mind that you're meant to be taking it easy.'

She giggled. 'Oh, smell that clean air!'

'And I'm a retired gentleman of leisure, as I have to keep telling myself.' He enjoyed a deep sigh of contentment. 'There's just one other thing, though, Helen: the title of Vee's book. Don't you think *Doors Closing* sounds a bit, well, final?'

'A bit, yes.'

He fixed his eyes on his beautiful lady.

30

Abbie's confession

Dear "Max",

I'm finding it difficult to leave this world I have created. But everything must come to an end, including the book. Doors open, doors close.

Now it's time for me to confess, reveal what's happened here, whether or not you ever get to read it. I have no way of finding out what has really happened in your life, but there are several things I might have written about if I'd wanted to continue this imaginary version of our lives. I might have moved on two years, for example, after your holiday; both of your daughters might have graduated, and perhaps "Grace" is training to be a doctor. Of course this might be true, but what I have written about you and your family is largely a figment of my imagination.

I could have left you all behind to focus on writing a book with no reference to anything at all you might recognise. Or the world I have invented here could go on turning longer, if I wanted it to, for good or ill. But I've decided that enough is enough; it is time to explain what's been going on. This particular world has to stop turning – now that I'm at a safe distance.

I doubt if I'll ever send this letter that I'm scribbling now: I don't even know where you live or how to get in touch with you now you've retired, Roy. That's how it should be, for a patient.

Obviously, I'm still around. I wrote about my own death and described what my own funeral might be like. Yes, I even wrote Newman's introduction. Of course, parts of the story, that is to say some of the details of my childhood, the existence of Aunt Mary, when you and I first met, my teaching career, how you became my doctor years later, the terrible life I had at Squaremile, and above all this life-changing illness – these are all real, as you know. I still have the white door with me but it has stayed closed for a while. For me, the fact that this particular door remains closed is a good thing.

I liked working with "Helen"; she was a good manager, but as far as I know, neither she nor you stepped in on my behalf. Of course, I didn't expect you to. The showdown and its repercussions were wishful thinking; Squaremile still exists and must be left to its own devices. In any case, it would be far too late to take any kind of action now. Let's just assume that this book gets published, and you get hold of a copy.

I hope you're both well and haven't suffered any major health issues like your fictional counterparts. Without their help, however, I would probably not be here, writing this in the new flat.

Yes, I *was* writing the book when I last saw you, but then you and Sonya ("Bella") decided I ought to spend some more time in Porteblanche. But I couldn't have handed over the manuscript at that appointment in August, because it was still just a collection of notes then. Besides, the idea of imagining your participation had not yet occurred to me.

By the time I came out of hospital again you'd left. I missed you and couldn't get used to not seeing you, so when I'd settled in my new place, I thought I'd create this other world, write about what *might* have happened, if you'd acted on my behalf. My life at Squaremile and the way I left were so chaotic that I just wanted it all sorted out; I couldn't think of anyone better qualified for the task than you. It seemed like a good way to structure what I wanted to say, and it somehow maintained your involvement in my progress.

So that's when *Doors Closing* came into being. I acquired

a computer and Len built me a desk with two chests and a stout work surface, so there was no excuse. I saw Sonya a few more times, but then she too left, disillusioned by changes within the NHS. But writing the book made me feel less alone.

Phisto died last year, at a ripe old age, and with him my last (and best) connection to Squaremile.

There was no baby, Roy. You don't need to worry on that score.

While I will never know how many other people might have been treated as I was, writing this book was my own way of coping, just as Newman said. Among other things, the book allowed me to explore my anger. But in the end, I hope you will see that I wrote it out of love for you. Remember those moments in the book when Max felt Vee's presence nearby? I was thinking about you as I wrote the scenes and wanted to be with you. That's all it was. Nothing more sinister. No ghosts or anything.

Dearest Roy. Enjoy your retirement, but don't forget the sunset and the champagne, Max!

Yours always,

Abbie (Vee)   *(Wie geht's?)*

Il n'y a pas d'amour de vivre sans désespoir de vivre.
ALBERT CAMUS

Translation of French
Used in the Text

Mais les souvenirs cheminent en nous alors que nous croyons les avoir fermement rélégués dans l'oubli.

JACQUELINE DE ROMILLY

But memories haunt us, even when we think we have resolutely consigned them to oblivion.

«Les plaies du coeur guérissent mal
Souventes fois même, salut!
Elles ne se referment plus.»

GEORGES BRASSENS

A wounded heart is slow to mend; oh, it's often the case that it never really heals.

Je suis dos.

This is a literal translation and means 'I am <u>back</u>' in the sense of 'spine.' To convey 'back', in the sense needed here, a verb such as 'returned' (revenu) would be needed.

«Si l'Eternel existe,
en fin de compte
Il voit qu'
je me conduis
guère plus mal
Que si j'avais la foi.»

GEORGES BRASSENS

If the Almighty exists, at the end of the day, He'll see that I'm behaving hardly any worse than if I believed.

Il n'y a pas d'amour de vivre sans désespoir de vivre.

ALBERT CAMUS

There is no love of life without despair of life.